Cram101 Textbook Outlines to accompany:

Sensation and Perception

Goldstein, 6th Edition

An Academic Internet Publishers (AIPI) publication (c) 2007.

Cram101 and Cram101.com are AIPI publications and services. All notes, highlights, reviews, and practice tests are prepared by AIPI for use in AIPI publications, all rights reserved.

You have a discounted membership at www.Cram101.com with this book.

Get all of the practice tests for the chapters of this textbook, and access in-depth reference material for writing essays and papers. Here is an example from a Cram101 Biology text:

When you need problem solving help with math, stats, and other disciplines, www.Cram101.com will walk through the formulas and solutions step by step.

With Cram101.com online, you also have access to extensive reference material.

You will nail those essays and papers. Here is an example from a Cram101 Biology text:

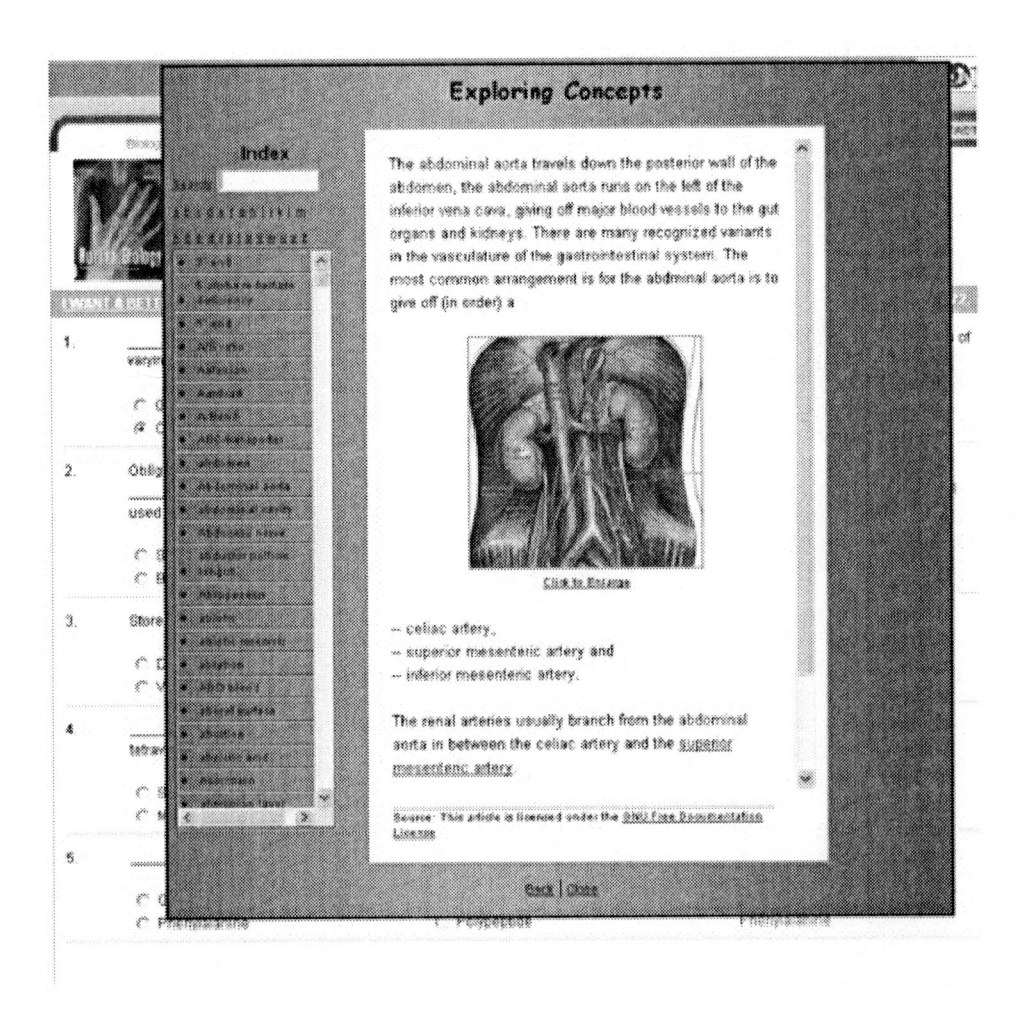

Visit **www.Cram101.com**, click Sign Up at the top of the screen, and enter DK73DW in the promo code box on the registration screen. Access to www.Cram101.com is normally $9.95, but because you have purchased this book, your access fee is only $4.95. Sign up and stop highlighting textbooks forever.

Learning System

Cram101 Textbook Outlines is a learning system. The notes in this book are the highlights of your textbook, you will never have to highlight a book again.

How to use this book. Take this book to class, it is your notebook for the lecture. The notes and highlights on the left hand side of the pages follow the outline and order of the textbook. All you have to do is follow along while your intructor presents the lecture. Circle the items emphasized in class and add other important information on the right side. With Cram101 Textbook Outlines you'll spend less time writing and more time listening. Learning becomes more efficient.

Cram101.com Online

Increase your studying efficiency by using Cram101.com's practice tests and online reference material. It is the perfect complement to Cram101 Textbook Outlines. Use self-teaching matching tests or simulate in-class testing with comprehensive multiple choice tests, or simply use Cram's true and false tests for quick review. Cram101.com even allows you to enter your in-class notes for an integrated studying format combining the textbook notes with your class notes.

Sensation and Perception
Goldstein, 6th

CONTENTS

1. Introduction to Perception 2
2. Receptors and Neural Processing 12
3. The Lateral Geniculate Nucleus and Striate Cortex 22
4. Higher-Level Visual Processing 28
5. Perceiving Objects 34
6. Perceiving Color 40
7. Perceiving Depth and Size 48
8. Perceiving Movement 54
9. Perception and Action 60
10. Sound, the Auditory System and Pitch Perception 64
11. Auditory Localization, Sound Quality and the Auditory Scene 72
12. Speech Perception 76
13. The Cutaneous Senses 82
14. The Chemical Senses 92
15. Perceptual Development 102
16. Clinical Aspects of Vision and Hearing 108

Chapter 1. Introduction to Perception

Information processing	Information processing is an approach to the goal of understanding human thinking. The essence of the approach is to see cognition as being essentially computational in nature, with mind being the software and the brain being the hardware.
Perception	Perception is the process of acquiring, interpreting, selecting, and organizing sensory information.
Senses	The senses are systems that consist of a sensory cell type that respond to a specific kind of physical energy, and that correspond to a defined region within the brain where the signals are received and interpreted.
Dyslexia	Dyslexia is a neurological disorder with biochemical and genetic markers. In its most common and apparent form, it is a disability in which a person's reading and/or writing ability is significantly lower than that which would be predicted by his or her general level of intelligence.
Chronic	Chronic refers to a relatively long duration, usually more than a few months.
Stimulus	A change in an environmental condition that elicits a response is a stimulus.
Transduction	Transduction in the nervous system typically refers to synaptic events wherein an electrical signal, known as an action potential, is converted into a chemical one via the release of neurotransmitters. Conversely, in sensory transduction a chemical or physical stimulus is transduced by sensory receptors into an electrical signal.
Receptor	A sensory receptor is a structure that recognizes a stimulus in the internal or external environment of an organism. In response to stimuli the sensory receptor initiates sensory transduction by creating graded potentials or action potentials in the same cell or in an adjacent one.
Retina	The retina is a thin layer of cells at the back of the eyeball. It is the part of the eye which converts light into nervous signals. The retina contains photoreceptor cells which receive the light; the resulting neural signals then undergo complex processing by other neurons of the retina, and are transformed into action potentials in retinal ganglion cells whose axons form the optic nerve.
Nervous system	The body's electrochemical communication circuitry, made up of billions of neurons is a nervous system.
Brain	The brain controls and coordinates most movement, behavior and homeostatic body functions such as heartbeat, blood pressure, fluid balance and body temperature. Functions of the brain are responsible for cognition, emotion, memory, motor learning and other sorts of learning. The brain is primarily made up of two types of cells: glia and neurons.
Neuron	The neuron is the primary cell of the nervous system. They are found in the brain, the spinal cord, in the nerves and ganglia of the peripheral nervous system. It is a specialized cell that conducts impulses through the nervous system and contains three major parts: cell body, dendrites, and an axon. It can have many dendrites but only one axon.
Affect	A subjective feeling or emotional tone often accompanied by bodily expressions noticeable to others is called affect.
Visual form agnosia	A variety of agnosia in which people can identify some elements of what they see but cannot perceive an object's shape is referred to as visual form agnosia.
Tumor	A tumor is an abnormal growth that when located in the brain can either be malignant and directly destroy brain tissue, or be benign and disrupt functioning by increasing intracranial pressure.
Attention	Attention is the cognitive process of selectively concentrating on one thing while ignoring other things. Psychologists have labeled three types of attention: sustained attention, selective attention, and divided attention.
Bottom-up processing	Using the parts of a pattern to recognize, or form an image of, the originating pattern is called bottom-up processing.
Top-down	In the Top-down model an overview of the system is formulated, without going into detail for any part

Chapter 1. Introduction to Perception

Chapter 1. Introduction to Perception

	of it. Each part of the system is then refined by designing it in more detail. Each new part may then be refined again, defining it in yet more detail until the entire specification is detailed enough to validate the Model.
American Psychological Association	The American Psychological Association is a professional organization representing psychology in the US. The mission statement is to "advance psychology as a science and profession and as a means of promoting health, education , and human welfare".
Neuroscience	A field that combines the work of psychologists, biologists, biochemists, medical researchers, and others in the study of the structure and function of the nervous system is neuroscience.
Society	The social sciences use the term society to mean a group of people that form a semi-closed (or semi-open) social system, in which most interactions are with other individuals belonging to the group.
Anatomy	Anatomy is the branch of biology that deals with the structure and organization of living things. It can be divided into animal anatomy (zootomy) and plant anatomy (phytonomy). Major branches of anatomy include comparative anatomy, histology, and human anatomy.
Apparent movement	Apparent movement is the perceived motion of an object when all that has been presented to the eyes is one or a series of stills.
Quantitative	A quantitative property is one that exists in a range of magnitudes, and can therefore be measured. Measurements of any particular quantitative property are expressed as as a specific quantity, referred to as a unit, multiplied by a number.
Physiology	The study of the functions and activities of living cells, tissues, and organs and of the physical and chemical phenomena involved is referred to as physiology.
Fechner	Fechner founded psychophysics or the scientific investigation of the functional relations of dependency between body and mind.
Method of limits	The method of limits is a psychophysical procedure for establishing sensory threshold values. The researcher increases or decreases the intensity of a stimulus until a subject can detect it 50 percent of the time.
Threshold	In general, a threshold is a fixed location or value where an abrupt change is observed. In the sensory modalities, it is the minimum amount of stimulus energy necessary to elicit a sensory response.
Method of constant stimuli	The method of constant stimuli is a psychophysical procedure for determining thresholds. The researcher presents stimuli of various magnitudes and asks the person to report their presence.
Difference threshold	Difference threshold refers to the minimal difference in intensity required between two sources of energy so that they will be perceived as being different 50 percent of the time.
Magnitude estimation	Magnitude estimation involves subjects attempting to report numerically the perceived intensity of sensation relative to a standard, where the standard is ascribed a specific numeric value either by the experimenter or subject.
Brightness	The dimension of visual sensation that is dependent on the intensity of light reflected from a surface and that corresponds to the amplitude of the light wave is called brightness.
Sensation	Sensation is the first stage in the chain of biochemical and neurologic events that begins with the impinging of a stimulus upon the receptor cells of a sensory organ, which then leads to perception, the mental state that is reflected in statements like "I see a uniformly blue wall."
Power law	Stevens' power law is a proposed relationship between the magnitude of a physical stimulus and its perceived intensity or strength. It is widely considered to supersede the Weber-Fechner law on the basis that it describes a wider range of sensations.
Nerve impulse	A nerve impulse is a change in the electric potential of a neuron; a wave of depolarization spreads

Chapter 1. Introduction to Perception

	along the neuron and causes the release of a neurotransmitter.
Aristotle	Aristotle can be credited with the development of the first theory of learning. He concluded that ideas were generated in consciousness based on four principlesof association: contiguity, similarity, contrast, and succession. In contrast to Plato, he believed that knowledge derived from sensory experience and was not inherited.
Emotion	An emotion is a mental states that arise spontaneously, rather than through conscious effort. They are often accompanied by physiological changes.
Sensory nerves	Sensory nerves bring impulses toward the central nervous system.
Nerve	A nerve is an enclosed, cable-like bundle of nerve fibers or axons, which includes the glia that ensheath the axons in myelin. Neurons are sometimes called nerve cells, though this term is technically imprecise since many neurons do not form nerves.
Optic nerve	The optic nerve is the nerve that transmits visual information from the retina to the brain. The optic nerve is composed of retinal ganglion cell axons and support cells.
Nucleus	In neuroanatomy, a cluster of cell bodies of neurons within the central nervous system is a nucleus.
Axon	An axon, or "nerve fiber," is a long slender projection of a nerve cell, or "neuron," which conducts electrical impulses away from the neuron's cell body or soma.
Adrian	Adrian formulated the all-or-nothing law of the neural cell in 1912 and measured the electric impulse of a single nerve 1926. According to the all-or-none law, a muscle or nerve fiber supplies the energy for the impulse and is completely discharged when excited at all.
Ion	An ion is an atom or group of atoms with a net electric charge. The energy required to detach an electron in its lowest energy state from an atom or molecule of a gas with less net electric charge is called the ionization potential, or ionization energy.
Microelectrode	An electrical wire so small that it can be used either to monitor the electrical activity of a single neuron or to stimulate activity within it is a microelectrode.
Electrode	Any device used to electrically stimulate nerve tissue or to record its activity is an electrode.
Resting potential	The resting potential of a cell is the membrane potential that would be maintained if there were no action potentials, synaptic potentials, or other active changes in the membrane potential. In most cells the resting potential has a negative value, which by convention means that there is excess negative charge inside compared to outside.
Action potential	The electrical impulse that provides the basis for the conduction of a neural impulse along an axon of a neuron is the action potential. When a biological cell or patch of membrane undergoes an action potential, or electrical excitation, the polarity of the transmembrane voltage swings rapidly from negative to positive and back.
Golgi	Golgi discovered a method of staining nervous tissue which would stain a limited number of cells at random, in their entirety. This enabled him to view the paths of nerve cells in the brain for the first time. He called his discovery the black reaction. It is now known universally as the Golgi stain.
Synapse	A synapse is specialized junction through which cells of the nervous system signal to one another and to non-neuronal cells such as muscles or glands.
Neurotransmitter	A neurotransmitter is a chemical that is used to relay, amplify and modulate electrical signals between a neurons and another cell.
Receptor site	A location on the dendrite of a receiving neuron that is tailored to receive a specific neurotransmitter is a receptor site.
Excitatory synapse	An excitatory synapse is where the neurotransmitter increases the likelihood that an action potential will occur, or increases the rate at which they are already occurring, in the neuron on which it acts.

Go to Cram101.com for the Practice Tests for this Chapter.

Chapter 1. Introduction to Perception

Chapter 1. Introduction to Perception

Inhibitory synapse	An inhibitory synapse is a synapse in which an action potential in the presynaptic cell decreases the probability of an action potential occurring in the postsynaptic cell.
Cerebral cortex	The cerebral cortex is the outermost layer of the cerebrum and has a grey color. It is made up of four lobes and it is involved in many complex brain functions including memory, perceptual awareness, "thinking", language and consciousness. The cerebral cortex receives sensory information from many different sensory organs eg: eyes, ears, etc. and processes the information.
Somatosensory cortex	The primary somatosensory cortex is across the central sulcus and behind the primary motor cortex configured to generally correspond with the arrangement of nearby motor cells related to specific body parts. It is the main sensory receptive area for the sense of touch.
Visual cortex	The visual cortex is the general term applied to both the primary visual cortex and the visual association area. Anatomically, the visual cortex occupies the entire occipital lobe, the inferior temporal lobe (IT), posterior parts of the parietal lobe, and a few small regions in the frontal lobe.
Parietal lobe	The parietal lobe is positioned above (superior to) the occipital lobe and behind (posterior to) the frontal lobe. It plays important roles in integrating sensory information from various senses, and in the manipulation of objects.
Temporal lobe	The temporal lobe is part of the cerebrum. It lies at the side of the brain, beneath the lateral or Sylvian fissure. Adjacent areas in the superior, posterior and lateral parts of the temporal lobe are involved in high-level auditory processing.
Frontal lobe	The frontal lobe comprises four major folds of cortical tissue: the precentral gyrus, superior gyrus and the middle gyrus of the frontal gyri, the inferior frontal gyrus. It has been found to play a part in impulse control, judgement, language, memory, motor function, problem solving, sexual behavior, socialization and spontaneity.
Olfaction	Olfaction, the sense of odor (smell), is the detection of chemicals dissolved in air. Smells are sensed by the olfactory epithelium located in the nose and processed by the olfactory system.
Positron emission tomography	Positron Emission Tomography measures emissions from radioactively labeled chemicals that have been injected into the bloodstream. The greatest benefit is that different compounds can show blood flow and oxygen and glucose metabolism in the tissues of the working brain.
Functional magnetic resonance imaging	Functional Magnetic Resonance Imaging describes the use of MRI to measure hemodynamic signals related to neural activity in the brain or spinal cord of humans or other animals. It is one of the most recently developed forms of brain imaging.
Neuroimaging	Neuroimaging comprises all invasive, minimally invasive, and non-invasive methods for obtaining structural and functional images of the nervous system's major subsystems: the brain, the peripheral nervous system, and the spinal cord.
Consciousness	The awareness of the sensations, thoughts, and feelings being experienced at a given moment is called consciousness.
Plasticity	The capacity for modification and change is referred to as plasticity.
Loudness	Loudness is the quality of a sound that is the primary psychological correlate of physical intensity. Loudness is often approximated by a power function with an exponent of 0.6 when plotted vs. sound pressure or 0.3 when plotted vs. sound intensity.
Reaction time	The amount of time required to respond to a stimulus is referred to as reaction time.
Absolute threshold	An absolute threshold is the minimum amount of stimulation required for a person to detect a stimulus fifty percent of the time.
Cell membrane	A component of every biological cell, the selectively permeable cell membrane is a thin and structured bilayer of phospholipid and protein molecules that envelopes the cell. It separates a cell's interior

Go to Cram101.com for the Practice Tests for this Chapter.

Chapter 1. Introduction to Perception

Chapter 1. Introduction to Perception

	from its surroundings and controls what moves in and out.
Lobes	The four major sections of the cerebral cortex: frontal, parietal, temporal, and occipital are called lobes.
Brain imaging	Brain imaging is a fairly recent discipline within medicine and neuroscience. Brain imaging falls into two broad categories -- structural imaging and functional imaging.

Chapter 1. Introduction to Perception

Chapter 2. Receptors and Neural Processing

Receptor	A sensory receptor is a structure that recognizes a stimulus in the internal or external environment of an organism. In response to stimuli the sensory receptor initiates sensory transduction by creating graded potentials or action potentials in the same cell or in an adjacent one.
Cones	Cones are photoreceptors that transmit sensations of color, function in bright light, and used in visual acuity. Infants prior to months of age can only distinguish green and red indicating the cones are not fully developed; they can see all of the colors by 2 months of
Rods	Rods are cylindrical shaped photoreceptors that are sensitive to the intensity of light. Rods require less light to function than cone cells, and therefore are the primary source of visual information at night.
Perception	Perception is the process of acquiring, interpreting, selecting, and organizing sensory information.
Thalamus	An area near the center of the brain involved in the relay of sensory information to the cortex and in the functions of sleep and attention is the thalamus.
Retina	The retina is a thin layer of cells at the back of the eyeball. It is the part of the eye which converts light into nervous signals. The retina contains photoreceptor cells which receive the light; the resulting neural signals then undergo complex processing by other neurons of the retina, and are transformed into action potentials in retinal ganglion cells whose axons form the optic nerve.
Neuron	The neuron is the primary cell of the nervous system. They are found in the brain, the spinal cord, in the nerves and ganglia of the peripheral nervous system. It is a specialized cell that conducts impulses through the nervous system and contains three major parts: cell body, dendrites, and an axon. It can have many dendrites but only one axon.
Stimulus	A change in an environmental condition that elicits a response is a stimulus.
Visible light	The part of the electromagnetic spectrum that stimulates the eye and produces visual sensations is called visible light.
Lateral geniculate nucleus	The lateral geniculate nucleus of the thalamus is a part of the brain, which is the primary processor of visual information, received from the retina, in the CNS.
Nerve	A nerve is an enclosed, cable-like bundle of nerve fibers or axons, which includes the glia that ensheath the axons in myelin. Neurons are sometimes called nerve cells, though this term is technically imprecise since many neurons do not form nerves.
Optic nerve	The optic nerve is the nerve that transmits visual information from the retina to the brain. The optic nerve is composed of retinal ganglion cell axons and support cells.
Striate cortex	The functionally defined primary visual cortex is approximately equivalent to the anatomically defined striate cortex located in the occipital lobe.
Occipital lobe	The occipital lobe is the smallest of four true lobes in the human brain. Located in the rearmost portion of the skull, the occipital lobe is part of the forebrain structure. It is the visual processing center.
Extrastriate cortex	The extrastriate cortex is the locus of mid-level vision. Neurons in the extrastriate cortex generally respond to visual stimuli within their receptive fields. These responses are modulated by extraretinal effects, like attention, working memory, and reward expectation.
Parietal lobe	The parietal lobe is positioned above (superior to) the occipital lobe and behind (posterior to) the frontal lobe. It plays important roles in integrating sensory information from various senses, and in the manipulation of objects.

Chapter 2. Receptors and Neural Processing

Chapter 2. Receptors and Neural Processing

Temporal lobe	The temporal lobe is part of the cerebrum. It lies at the side of the brain, beneath the lateral or Sylvian fissure. Adjacent areas in the superior, posterior and lateral parts of the temporal lobe are involved in high-level auditory processing.
Epithelium	Epithelium is a tissue composed of a layer of cells. Epithelium can be found lining internal or external (e.g. skin) free surfaces of the body. Functions of epithelial cells include secretion, absorption and protection.
Fovea	The fovea, a part of the eye, is a spot located in the center of the macula. The fovea is responsible for sharp central vision, which is necessary in humans for reading, watching television or movies, driving, and any activity where visual detail is of primary importance.
Depression	In everyday language depression refers to any downturn in mood, which may be relatively transitory and perhaps due to something trivial. This is differentiated from Clinical depression which is marked by symptoms that last two weeks or more and are so severe that they interfere with daily living.
Shaping	The concept of reinforcing successive, increasingly accurate approximations to a target behavior is called shaping. The target behavior is broken down into a hierarchy of elemental steps, each step more sophisticated then the last. By successively reinforcing each of the the elemental steps, a form of differential reinforcement, until that step is learned while extinguishing the step below, the target behavior is gradually achieved.
Cornea	The cornea is the transparent front part of the eye that covers the iris, pupil, and anterior chamber and provides most of an eye's optical power. Together with the lens, the cornea refracts light and consequently helps the eye to focus.
Accommodation	Piaget's developmental process of accommodation is the modification of currently held schemes or new schemes so that new information inconsistent with the existing schemes can be integrated and understood.
Ganglion cell	A ganglion cell is a type of neuron located in the retina of the eye that receives visual information from photoreceptors via various intermediate cells such as bipolar cells, amacrine cells, and horizontal cells. Retinal ganglion cells' axons are myelinated.
Blind spot	In anatomy, the blind spot is the region of the retina where the optic nerve and blood vessels pass through to connect to the back of the eye. Since there are no light receptors there, a part of the field of vision is not perceived.
Horizontal cells	Horizontal cells are the laterally interconnecting neurons in the outer plexiform layer of the retina.
Ganglion	A ganglion is a tissue mass that contains the dendrites and cell bodies (or "somas") of nerve cells, in most case ones belonging to the peripheral nervous system. Within the central nervous system such a mass is often called a nucleus.
Photon	A photon is a quantum of the electromagnetic field, for instance light. In some respects a photon acts as a particle, for instance when registered by the light sensitive device in a camera. It also acts like a wave, as when passing through the optics in a camera.
Absolute threshold	An absolute threshold is the minimum amount of stimulation required for a person to detect a stimulus fifty percent of the time.
Protein	A protein is a complex, high-molecular-weight organic compound that consists of amino acids joined by peptide bonds. It is essential to the structure and function of all living cells and viruses. Many are enzymes or subunits of enzymes.
Physiology	The study of the functions and activities of living cells, tissues, and organs and of the physical and chemical phenomena involved is referred to as physiology.

Chapter 2. Receptors and Neural Processing

Chapter 2. Receptors and Neural Processing

Enzyme	An enzyme is a protein that catalyzes, or speeds up, a chemical reaction. Enzymes are essential to sustain life because most chemical reactions in biological cells would occur too slowly, or would lead to different products, without enzymes.
Dark adaptation	Dark adaptation is the tendency for the peak sensitivity of the human eye to shift toward the blue end of the color spectrum at low illumination levels.
Stages	Stages represent relatively discrete periods of time in which functioning is qualitatively different from functioning at other periods.
Adaptation	Adaptation is a lowering of sensitivity to a stimulus following prolonged exposure to that stimulus. Behavioral adaptations are special ways a particular organism behaves to survive in its natural habitat.
Fixation	Fixation in abnormal psychology is the state where an individual becomes obsessed with an attachment to another human, animal or inanimate object. Fixation in vision refers to maintaining the gaze in a constant direction. .
Monochromat	A monochromat is an organism that is truly color blind. That is, the perceptual effect of any arbitrarily chosen light from its visible spectrum can be matched by any pure spectral light. Monochromats can only see shades of black, gray and white.
Transduction	Transduction in the nervous system typically refers to synaptic events wherein an electrical signal, known as an action potential, is converted into a chemical one via the release of neurotransmitters. Conversely, in sensory transduction a chemical or physical stimulus is transduced by sensory receptors into an electrical signal.
Visible spectrum	The narrow band of electromagnetic waves, 380-760 nm in length, that are visible to the human eye is referred to as the visible spectrum.
Threshold	In general, a threshold is a fixed location or value where an abrupt change is observed. In the sensory modalities, it is the minimum amount of stimulus energy necessary to elicit a sensory response.
Synapse	A synapse is specialized junction through which cells of the nervous system signal to one another and to non-neuronal cells such as muscles or glands.
Nervous system	The body's electrochemical communication circuitry, made up of billions of neurons is a nervous system.
Cone vision	Cone vision refers to the high-acuity color vision that occurs in moderate to bright light and is mediated by receptor cones in the retina. It is also called photopic or bright-light vision.
Rod vision	Rod vision refers to the low-acuity, high-sensitivity, noncolor vision that occurs in dim light and is mediated by rods in the retina of the eye.
Attention	Attention is the cognitive process of selectively concentrating on one thing while ignoring other things. Psychologists have labeled three types of attention: sustained attention, selective attention, and divided attention.
Visual acuity	Visual acuity is the eye's ability to detect fine details and is the quantitative measure of the eye's ability to see an in-focus image at a certain distance.
Peripheral vision	Peripheral vision is that part of vision that occurs outside the very center of gaze. Peripheral vision is weak in humans, especially at distinguishing color and shape. This is because the density of receptor cells on the retina is greatest at the center and lowest at the edges
Excitatory synapse	An excitatory synapse is where the neurotransmitter increases the likelihood that an action potential will occur, or increases the rate at which they are already occurring, in the

Go to Cram101.com for the Practice Tests for this Chapter.

Chapter 2. Receptors and Neural Processing

neuron on which it acts.

Inhibitory synapse	An inhibitory synapse is a synapse in which an action potential in the presynaptic cell decreases the probability of an action potential occurring in the postsynaptic cell.
Affect	A subjective feeling or emotional tone often accompanied by bodily expressions noticeable to others is called affect.
Receptive field	The receptive field of a sensory neuron is a region of sensitivity in which the presence of a stimulus will alter the firing of that neuron.
Amacrine cells	Amacrine cells are interneurons in the retina which operate at the Inner Plexiform Layer (IPL), the second synaptic retinal layer where bipolar cells and ganglion cells synapse. Functionally, they are responsible for complex processing of the retinal image, specifically adjusting image brightness and, by integrating sequential activation of neurons, detecting motion.
Axon	An axon, or "nerve fiber," is a long slender projection of a nerve cell, or "neuron," which conducts electrical impulses away from the neuron's cell body or soma.
Electrode	Any device used to electrically stimulate nerve tissue or to record its activity is an electrode.
Bipolar cell	As a part of the retina, the bipolar cell exists between photoreceptors and ganglion cells. Bipolar cells are so-named as they have a central body from which two sets of processes arise. At one end, they form synapses with either a single cone cell, or a number of rod cells. At the other end, they form synapses with ganglion cells, which fire action potentials along the optic nerve (cranial nerve II). They effectively transfer information from rods and cones to ganglion cells.
Brightness	The dimension of visual sensation that is dependent on the intensity of light reflected from a surface and that corresponds to the amplitude of the light wave is called brightness.
Brain	The brain controls and coordinates most movement, behavior and homeostatic body functions such as heartbeat, blood pressure, fluid balance and body temperature. Functions of the brain are responsible for cognition, emotion, memory, motor learning and other sorts of learning. The brain is primarily made up of two types of cells: glia and neurons.
Nucleus	In neuroanatomy, a cluster of cell bodies of neurons within the central nervous system is a nucleus.
Senses	The senses are systems that consist of a sensory cell type that respond to a specific kind of physical energy, and that correspond to a defined region within the brain where the signals are received and interpreted.
Mach band	A Mach band is an optical illusion. It is the region encircling a bright light which in visual perception appears lighter or darker than its surroundings, in a zone where the luminance increases or decreases rapidly.
Illusion	An illusion is a distortion of a sensory perception.
Contrast effect	A contrast effect is the enhancement or diminishment, relative to normal, of a perception and related performance as a result of immediately previous or simultaneous exposure to a stimulus of lesser or greater value in the same dimension.
Functional magnetic resonance imaging	Functional Magnetic Resonance Imaging describes the use of MRI to measure hemodynamic signals related to neural activity in the brain or spinal cord of humans or other animals. It is one of the most recently developed forms of brain imaging.
Receptor site	A location on the dendrite of a receiving neuron that is tailored to receive a specific

Go to Cram101.com for the Practice Tests for this Chapter.

Chapter 2. Receptors and Neural Processing

neurotransmitter is a receptor site.

Chapter 3. The Lateral Geniculate Nucleus and Striate Cortex

Retina	The retina is a thin layer of cells at the back of the eyeball. It is the part of the eye which converts light into nervous signals. The retina contains photoreceptor cells which receive the light; the resulting neural signals then undergo complex processing by other neurons of the retina, and are transformed into action potentials in retinal ganglion cells whose axons form the optic nerve.
Receptor	A sensory receptor is a structure that recognizes a stimulus in the internal or external environment of an organism. In response to stimuli the sensory receptor initiates sensory transduction by creating graded potentials or action potentials in the same cell or in an adjacent one.
Receptive field	The receptive field of a sensory neuron is a region of sensitivity in which the presence of a stimulus will alter the firing of that neuron.
Ganglion cell	A ganglion cell is a type of neuron located in the retina of the eye that receives visual information from photoreceptors via various intermediate cells such as bipolar cells, amacrine cells, and horizontal cells. Retinal ganglion cells' axons are myelinated.
Optic nerve	The optic nerve is the nerve that transmits visual information from the retina to the brain. The optic nerve is composed of retinal ganglion cell axons and support cells.
Axon	An axon, or "nerve fiber," is a long slender projection of a nerve cell, or "neuron," which conducts electrical impulses away from the neuron's cell body or soma.
Lateral geniculate nucleus	The lateral geniculate nucleus of the thalamus is a part of the brain, which is the primary processor of visual information, received from the retina, in the CNS.
Visual cortex	The visual cortex is the general term applied to both the primary visual cortex and the visual association area. Anatomically, the visual cortex occupies the entire occipital lobe, the inferior temporal lobe (IT), posterior parts of the parietal lobe, and a few small regions in the frontal lobe.
Neuron	The neuron is the primary cell of the nervous system. They are found in the brain, the spinal cord, in the nerves and ganglia of the peripheral nervous system. It is a specialized cell that conducts impulses through the nervous system and contains three major parts: cell body, dendrites, and an axon. It can have many dendrites but only one axon.
Brain stem	The brain stem is the stalk of the brain below the cerebral hemispheres. It is the major route for communication between the forebrain and the spinal cord and peripheral nerves. It also controls various functions including respiration, regulation of heart rhythms, and primary aspects of sound localization.
Thalamus	An area near the center of the brain involved in the relay of sensory information to the cortex and in the functions of sleep and attention is the thalamus.
Nucleus	In neuroanatomy, a cluster of cell bodies of neurons within the central nervous system is a nucleus.
Excitatory synapse	An excitatory synapse is where the neurotransmitter increases the likelihood that an action potential will occur, or increases the rate at which they are already occurring, in the neuron on which it acts.
Right hemisphere	The brain is divided into left and right cerebral hemispheres. The right hemisphere of the cortex controls the left side of the body.
Left hemisphere	The left hemisphere of the cortex controls the right side of the body, coordinates complex movements, and, in 95% of people, controls the production of speech and written language.
Striate cortex	The functionally defined primary visual cortex is approximately equivalent to the

Go to **Cram101.com** for the Practice Tests for this Chapter.

Chapter 3. The Lateral Geniculate Nucleus and Striate Cortex

	anatomically defined striate cortex located in the occipital lobe.
Brain	The brain controls and coordinates most movement, behavior and homeostatic body functions such as heartbeat, blood pressure, fluid balance and body temperature. Functions of the brain are responsible for cognition, emotion, memory, motor learning and other sorts of learning. The brain is primarily made up of two types of cells: glia and neurons.
Synapse	A synapse is specialized junction through which cells of the nervous system signal to one another and to non-neuronal cells such as muscles or glands.
Electrode	Any device used to electrically stimulate nerve tissue or to record its activity is an electrode.
Information processing	Information processing is an approach to the goal of understanding human thinking. The essence of the approach is to see cognition as being essentially computational in nature, with mind being the software and the brain being the hardware.
Nerve	A nerve is an enclosed, cable-like bundle of nerve fibers or axons, which includes the glia that ensheath the axons in myelin. Neurons are sometimes called nerve cells, though this term is technically imprecise since many neurons do not form nerves.
Nervous system	The body's electrochemical communication circuitry, made up of billions of neurons is a nervous system.
Adaptation	Adaptation is a lowering of sensitivity to a stimulus following prolonged exposure to that stimulus. Behavioral adaptations are special ways a particular organism behaves to survive in its natural habitat.
Physiology	The study of the functions and activities of living cells, tissues, and organs and of the physical and chemical phenomena involved is referred to as physiology.
Stimulus	A change in an environmental condition that elicits a response is a stimulus.
Simple cell	A neuron in the striate cortex that is maximally sensitive to the position and orientation of edges in the receptive field is called a simple cell.
Nerve impulse	A nerve impulse is a change in the electric potential of a neuron; a wave of depolarization spreads along the neuron and causes the release of a neurotransmitter.
Psychophysics	Psychophysics refers to the study of the mathematical relationship between the physical aspects of stimuli and our psychological experience of them.
Perception	Perception is the process of acquiring, interpreting, selecting, and organizing sensory information.
Amplitude	Amplitude is a nonnegative scalar measure of a wave's magnitude of oscillation.
Threshold	In general, a threshold is a fixed location or value where an abrupt change is observed. In the sensory modalities, it is the minimum amount of stimulus energy necessary to elicit a sensory response.
Affect	A subjective feeling or emotional tone often accompanied by bodily expressions noticeable to others is called affect.
Spatial frequency	The number of repetitions, per unit distance, of the repeating elements of the image of a pattern on the retina of the eye is called the spatial frequency.
Analyzer	Pavlov's name for a specialized part of the nervous system is Analyzer, which controls the reactions of the organism to changing external conditions. It consists of sense receptors, the sensory pathway to the cortex, and the area of the cortex where the sensory activity is projected.

Go to **Cram101.com** for the Practice Tests for this Chapter.

Chapter 3. The Lateral Geniculate Nucleus and Striate Cortex

Chapter 3. The Lateral Geniculate Nucleus and Striate Cortex

Feature detector	A feature detector is sensory system that is highly attuned to a specific stimulus pattern. They are nerve cells in the brain that respond to specific features of the stimulus, such as shape, angle, or movement.
Fovea	The fovea, a part of the eye, is a spot located in the center of the macula. The fovea is responsible for sharp central vision, which is necessary in humans for reading, watching television or movies, driving, and any activity where visual detail is of primary importance.
Cones	Cones are photoreceptors that transmit sensations of color, function in bright light, and used in visual acuity. Infants prior to months of age can only distinguish green and red indicating the cones are not fully developed; they can see all of the colors by 2 months of
Microelectrode	An electrical wire so small that it can be used either to monitor the electrical activity of a single neuron or to stimulate activity within it is a microelectrode.
Glucose	Glucose, a simple monosaccharide sugar, is one of the most important carbohydrates and is used as a source of energy in animals and plants. Glucose is one of the main products of photosynthesis and starts respiration.
Plasticity	The capacity for modification and change is referred to as plasticity.
Learning	Learning is a relatively permanent change in behavior that results from experience. Thus, to attribute a behavioral change to learning, the change must be relatively permanent and must result from experience.
Hebb	Hebb demonstrated that the rearing of rats in an enriched environment could alter neural development and that sensory - neural connections were shaped by experience. He is famous for developing the concept of neural nets. He also believed that learning early in life is of the incremental variety, whereas later it is cognitive, insightful, and more all-or-none.
Astigmatism	Astigmatism is a refraction error of the eye characterized by an aspherical cornea in which one axis of corneal steepness is greater than the perpendicular axis.
Somatosensory cortex	The primary somatosensory cortex is across the central sulcus and behind the primary motor cortex configured to generally correspond with the arrangement of nearby motor cells related to specific body parts. It is the main sensory receptive area for the sense of touch.
Auditory system	The auditory system is the sensory system for the sense of hearing. On its path from the outside world to the forebrain, sound information is preserved and modified in many ways. It changes media twice, first from air to fluid, then from fluid to action potentials.
Somatosensory	Somatosensory system consists of the various sensory receptors that trigger the experiences labelled as touch or pressure, temperature, pain, and the sensations of muscle movement and joint position including posture, movement, and facial expression.
Senses	The senses are systems that consist of a sensory cell type that respond to a specific kind of physical energy, and that correspond to a defined region within the brain where the signals are received and interpreted.
Mand	The mand is verbal behavior whose form is controlled by states of deprivation and aversion; it is often said to "specify its own reinforcer." What this means loosely is that the function of a mand is to request or to obtain what is wanted.

Chapter 4. Higher-Level Visual Processing

Striate cortex	The functionally defined primary visual cortex is approximately equivalent to the anatomically defined striate cortex located in the occipital lobe.
Neuron	The neuron is the primary cell of the nervous system. They are found in the brain, the spinal cord, in the nerves and ganglia of the peripheral nervous system. It is a specialized cell that conducts impulses through the nervous system and contains three major parts: cell body, dendrites, and an axon. It can have many dendrites but only one axon.
Perception	Perception is the process of acquiring, interpreting, selecting, and organizing sensory information.
Extrastriate cortex	The extrastriate cortex is the locus of mid-level vision. Neurons in the extrastriate cortex generally respond to visual stimuli within their receptive fields. These responses are modulated by extraretinal effects, like attention, working memory, and reward expectation.
Visual perception	Visual perception is one of the senses, consisting of the ability to detect light and interpret it. Vision has a specific sensory system.
Cerebral cortex	The cerebral cortex is the outermost layer of the cerebrum and has a grey color. It is made up of four lobes and it is involved in many complex brain functions including memory, perceptual awareness, "thinking", language and consciousness. The cerebral cortex receives sensory information from many different sensory organs eg: eyes, ears, etc. and processes the information.
Parietal lobe	The parietal lobe is positioned above (superior to) the occipital lobe and behind (posterior to) the frontal lobe. It plays important roles in integrating sensory information from various senses, and in the manipulation of objects.
Frontal lobe	The frontal lobe comprises four major folds of cortical tissue: the precentral gyrus, superior gyrus and the middle gyrus of the frontal gyri, the inferior frontal gyrus. It has been found to play a part in impulse control, judgement, language, memory, motor function, problem solving, sexual behavior, socialization and spontaneity.
Physiology	The study of the functions and activities of living cells, tissues, and organs and of the physical and chemical phenomena involved is referred to as physiology.
Stimulus	A change in an environmental condition that elicits a response is a stimulus.
Synapse	A synapse is specialized junction through which cells of the nervous system signal to one another and to non-neuronal cells such as muscles or glands.
Temporal lobe	The temporal lobe is part of the cerebrum. It lies at the side of the brain, beneath the lateral or Sylvian fissure. Adjacent areas in the superior, posterior and lateral parts of the temporal lobe are involved in high-level auditory processing.
Brain	The brain controls and coordinates most movement, behavior and homeostatic body functions such as heartbeat, blood pressure, fluid balance and body temperature. Functions of the brain are responsible for cognition, emotion, memory, motor learning and other sorts of learning. The brain is primarily made up of two types of cells: glia and neurons.
Discrimination	In Learning theory, discrimination refers the ability to distinguish between a conditioned stimulus and other stimuli. It can be brought about by extensive training or differential reinforcement. In social terms, it is the denial of privileges to a person or a group on the basis of prejudice.
Where pathway	The where pathway refers to the upper portions of the occipital and parietal lobes of the cortex. Damage interferes with the ability to locate objects and guide one's own actions.
Mand	The mand is verbal behavior whose form is controlled by states of deprivation and aversion; it is often said to "specify its own reinforcer." What this means loosely is that the

Go to **Cram101.com** for the Practice Tests for this Chapter.

Chapter 4. Higher-Level Visual Processing

	function of a mand is to request or to obtain what is wanted.
Dorsal stream	The dorsal stream is a pathway for visual information which flows through the visual cortex, the part of the brain which provides visual processing. It is involved in spatial awareness: recognizing where objects are in space.
Ventral stream	The primate visual system consists of about thirty areas of the cerebral cortex called the visual cortex. The visual cortex is divided into the ventral stream and the dorsal stream. The ventral stream is associated with object recognition and form representation.
Neuropsychology	Neuropsychology is a branch of psychology that aims to understand how the structure and function of the brain relates to specific psychological processes.
Dissociation	Dissociation is a psychological state or condition in which certain thoughts, emotions, sensations, or memories are separated from the rest.
Reasoning	Reasoning is the act of using reason to derive a conclusion from certain premises. There are two main methods to reach a conclusion, deductive reasoning and inductive reasoning.
Threshold	In general, a threshold is a fixed location or value where an abrupt change is observed. In the sensory modalities, it is the minimum amount of stimulus energy necessary to elicit a sensory response.
Modularity of mind	Modularity of Mind is the notion that a mind may be composed of modules, at least in part. Proponents believe this view is implied by Noam Chomsky's concept of a universal, generative grammar. Such features of language imply there's an underlying "language acquisition device" structure in the brain.
Correlation	A statistical technique for determining the degree of association between two or more variables is referred to as correlation.
Coding	In senation, coding is the process by which information about the quality and quantity of a stimulus is preserved in the pattern of action potentials sent through sensory neurons to the central nervous system.
Retina	The retina is a thin layer of cells at the back of the eyeball. It is the part of the eye which converts light into nervous signals. The retina contains photoreceptor cells which receive the light; the resulting neural signals then undergo complex processing by other neurons of the retina, and are transformed into action potentials in retinal ganglion cells whose axons form the optic nerve.
Nervous system	The body's electrochemical communication circuitry, made up of billions of neurons is a nervous system.
Natural selection	Natural selection is a process by which biological populations are altered over time, as a result of the propagation of heritable traits that affect the capacity of individual organisms to survive and reproduce.
Learning	Learning is a relatively permanent change in behavior that results from experience. Thus, to attribute a behavioral change to learning, the change must be relatively permanent and must result from experience.
Plasticity	The capacity for modification and change is referred to as plasticity.
Affect	A subjective feeling or emotional tone often accompanied by bodily expressions noticeable to others is called affect.
Binocular rivalry	Binocular rivalry is a phenomenon of visual perception in which perception alternates between different images presented to each eye. When one image is presented to one eye and a very different image is presented to the other, instead of the two images being seen superimposed, one image is seen for a few moments, then the other.

Chapter 4. Higher-Level Visual Processing

Attention	Attention is the cognitive process of selectively concentrating on one thing while ignoring other things. Psychologists have labeled three types of attention: sustained attention, selective attention, and divided attention.
Receptor	A sensory receptor is a structure that recognizes a stimulus in the internal or external environment of an organism. In response to stimuli the sensory receptor initiates sensory transduction by creating graded potentials or action potentials in the same cell or in an adjacent one.
Receptive field	The receptive field of a sensory neuron is a region of sensitivity in which the presence of a stimulus will alter the firing of that neuron.
Selective attention	Selective attention is a type of attention which involves focusing on a specific aspect of a scene while ignoring other aspects.
Fixation	Fixation in abnormal psychology is the state where an individual becomes obsessed with an attachment to another human, animal or inanimate object. Fixation in vision refers to maintaining the gaze in a constant direction. .
Hypothesis	A specific statement about behavior or mental processes that is testable through research is a hypothesis.
Electrode	Any device used to electrically stimulate nerve tissue or to record its activity is an electrode.
Synchrony	In child development, synchrony is the carefully coordinated interaction between the parent and the child or adolescent in which, often unknowingly, they are attuned to each other's behavior.
Senses	The senses are systems that consist of a sensory cell type that respond to a specific kind of physical energy, and that correspond to a defined region within the brain where the signals are received and interpreted.
Tactile	Pertaining to the sense of touch is referred to as tactile.
Evolution	Commonly used to refer to gradual change, evolution is the change in the frequency of alleles within a population from one generation to the next. This change may be caused by different mechanisms, including natural selection, genetic drift, or changes in population (gene flow).
Modulation	Modulation is the process of varying a carrier signal, typically a sinusoidal signal, in order to use that signal to convey information.
Motion perception	Motion perception is the process of inferring the "true" velocity and direction of motion in a visual scene given some visual input.
Gyrus	A gyrus is a ridge on the cerebral cortex. It is generally surrounded by one or more sulci.

Chapter 4. Higher-Level Visual Processing

Chapter 5. Perceiving Objects

Perception	Perception is the process of acquiring, interpreting, selecting, and organizing sensory information.
Structuralism	The school of psychology that argues that the mind consists of three basic elements sensations, feelings, and images which combine to form experience is structuralism-- a term coined by Titchener. They were associationists in that they believed that complex ideas were made up of simpler ideas that were combined in accordance with the laws of association.
Wundt	Wundt, considered the father of experimental psychology, created the first laboratory in psychology in 1879. His methodology was based on introspection and his body of work founded the school of thought called Voluntarism.
Gestalt psychology	According to Gestalt psychology, people naturally organize their perceptions according to certain patterns. The tendency is to organize perceptions into wholes and to integrate separate stimuli into meaningful patterns.
Nervous system	The body's electrochemical communication circuitry, made up of billions of neurons is a nervous system.
Brain	The brain controls and coordinates most movement, behavior and homeostatic body functions such as heartbeat, blood pressure, fluid balance and body temperature. Functions of the brain are responsible for cognition, emotion, memory, motor learning and other sorts of learning. The brain is primarily made up of two types of cells: glia and neurons.
Wertheimer	His discovery of the phi phenomenon concerning the illusion of motion gave rise to the influential school of Gestalt psychology. In the latter part of his life, Wertheimer directed much of his attention to the problem of learning.
Illusion	An illusion is a distortion of a sensory perception.
Sensation	Sensation is the first stage in the chain of biochemical and neurologic events that begins with the impinging of a stimulus upon the receptor cells of a sensory organ, which then leads to perception, the mental state that is reflected in statements like "I see a uniformly blue wall."
Apparent movement	Apparent movement is the perceived motion of an object when all that has been presented to the eyes is one or a series of stills.
Stimulus	A change in an environmental condition that elicits a response is a stimulus.
Retina	The retina is a thin layer of cells at the back of the eyeball. It is the part of the eye which converts light into nervous signals. The retina contains photoreceptor cells which receive the light; the resulting neural signals then undergo complex processing by other neurons of the retina, and are transformed into action potentials in retinal ganglion cells whose axons form the optic nerve.
Law of Pragnanz	The most basic rule of gestalt is the law of pragnanz. This law says that we try to experience things in as good a gestalt way as possible. In this sense, "good" can mean several things, such as regular, orderly, simplistic, symmetrical, etc.
Hue	A hue refers to the gradation of color within the optical spectrum, or visible spectrum, of light. Hue may also refer to a particular color within this spectrum, as defined by its dominant wavelength, or the central tendency of its combined wavelengths.
Law of common fate	The Gestalt Law of Common Fate argues that elements having the apparent same moving direction are seen as a unit.
Heuristic	A heuristic is a simple, efficient rule of thumb proposed to explain how people make decisions, come to judgments and solve problems, typically when facing complex problems or incomplete information. These rules work well under most circumstances, but in certain cases

Go to **Cram101.com** for the Practice Tests for this Chapter.

Chapter 5. Perceiving Objects

Chapter 5. Perceiving Objects

	lead to systematic cognitive biases.
Algorithm	A systematic procedure for solving a problem that works invariably when it is correctly applied is called an algorithm.
Neuron	The neuron is the primary cell of the nervous system. They are found in the brain, the spinal cord, in the nerves and ganglia of the peripheral nervous system. It is a specialized cell that conducts impulses through the nervous system and contains three major parts: cell body, dendrites, and an axon. It can have many dendrites but only one axon.
Evolution	Commonly used to refer to gradual change, evolution is the change in the frequency of alleles within a population from one generation to the next. This change may be caused by different mechanisms, including natural selection, genetic drift, or changes in population (gene flow).
Learning	Learning is a relatively permanent change in behavior that results from experience. Thus, to attribute a behavioral change to learning, the change must be relatively permanent and must result from experience.
Problem solving	An attempt to find an appropriate way of attaining a goal when the goal is not readily available is called problem solving.
Infancy	The developmental period that extends from birth to 18 or 24 months is called infancy.
Principles of Perceptual Organization	The Gestalt psychologists outlined what seemed to be several fundamental and universal principles of perceptual organization which described the principles by which the elements of perception are organized into configurations .
Connectedness	Connectedness, according to Cooper, consists of two dimensions: mutuality and permeability. Connectedness involves processes that link the self to others, as seen in acknowledgment of, respect for, and responsiveness to others.
Synchrony	In child development, synchrony is the carefully coordinated interaction between the parent and the child or adolescent in which, often unknowingly, they are attuned to each other's behavior.
Quantitative	A quantitative property is one that exists in a range of magnitudes, and can therefore be measured. Measurements of any particular quantitative property are expressed as as a specific quantity, referred to as a unit, multiplied by a number.
Discrimination	In Learning theory, discrimination refers the ability to distinguish between a conditioned stimulus and other stimuli. It can be brought about by extensive training or differential reinforcement. In social terms, it is the denial of privileges to a person or a group on the basis of prejudice.
Reaction time	The amount of time required to respond to a stimulus is referred to as reaction time.
Affect	A subjective feeling or emotional tone often accompanied by bodily expressions noticeable to others is called affect.
Homogeneous	In biology homogeneous has a meaning similar to its meaning in mathematics. Generally it means "the same" or "of the same quality or general property".
Extrastriate cortex	The extrastriate cortex is the locus of mid-level vision. Neurons in the extrastriate cortex generally respond to visual stimuli within their receptive fields. These responses are modulated by extraretinal effects, like attention, working memory, and reward expectation.
Physiology	The study of the functions and activities of living cells, tissues, and organs and of the physical and chemical phenomena involved is referred to as physiology.
Gestalt laws of organization	Gestalt laws of organization are a series of principles that describe how we organize bits and pieces of information into meaningful wholes.

Go to **Cram101.com** for the Practice Tests for this Chapter.

Chapter 5. Perceiving Objects

Chapter 5. Perceiving Objects

Figure-ground	The Gestalt principle of Figure-ground states that there is an innate tendency to perceive one aspect of an event as the figure or foreground and the other as the ground or the background.
Stages	Stages represent relatively discrete periods of time in which functioning is qualitatively different from functioning at other periods.
Brightness	The dimension of visual sensation that is dependent on the intensity of light reflected from a surface and that corresponds to the amplitude of the light wave is called brightness.
Attention	Attention is the cognitive process of selectively concentrating on one thing while ignoring other things. Psychologists have labeled three types of attention: sustained attention, selective attention, and divided attention.
Ion	An ion is an atom or group of atoms with a net electric charge. The energy required to detach an electron in its lowest energy state from an atom or molecule of a gas with less net electric charge is called the ionization potential, or ionization energy.
Construct	A generalized concept, such as anxiety or gravity, is a construct.
Invariance	Invariance is the property of perception whereby simple geometrical objects are recognized independent of rotation, translation, and scale, as well as several other variations such as elastic deformations, different lighting, and different component features.
Hippocampus	The hippocampus is a part of the brain located inside the temporal lobe. It forms a part of the limbic system and plays a part in memory and navigation.
Receptor	A sensory receptor is a structure that recognizes a stimulus in the internal or external environment of an organism. In response to stimuli the sensory receptor initiates sensory transduction by creating graded potentials or action potentials in the same cell or in an adjacent one.
Top-down	In the Top-down model an overview of the system is formulated, without going into detail for any part of it. Each part of the system is then refined by designing it in more detail. Each new part may then be refined again, defining it in yet more detail until the entire specification is detailed enough to validate the Model.
Theories	Theories are logically self-consistent models or frameworks describing the behavior of a certain natural or social phenomenon. They are broad explanations and predictions concerning phenomena of interest.
Chemical senses	Chemical senses include smell and taste.
Brain imaging	Brain imaging is a fairly recent discipline within medicine and neuroscience. Brain imaging falls into two broad categories -- structural imaging and functional imaging.
Projection	Attributing one's own undesirable thoughts, impulses, traits, or behaviors to others is referred to as projection.
Occlusion	The monocular depth cue occlusion is the blocking of sight of objects by other objects. It creates a "ranking" of nearness, and does not give any insight as to actual distances. In the absence of color or binocular vision, it often serves as the method of last resort for rudimentary depth perception.
Plasticity	The capacity for modification and change is referred to as plasticity.
Senses	The senses are systems that consist of a sensory cell type that respond to a specific kind of physical energy, and that correspond to a defined region within the brain where the signals are received and interpreted.

Chapter 5. Perceiving Objects

Chapter 6. Perceiving Color

Color blindness	Color blindness in humans is the inability to perceive differences between some or all colors that other people can distinguish. It is most often of genetic nature, but may also occur because of eye, nerve, or brain damage, or due to exposure to certain chemicals.
Receptor	A sensory receptor is a structure that recognizes a stimulus in the internal or external environment of an organism. In response to stimuli the sensory receptor initiates sensory transduction by creating graded potentials or action potentials in the same cell or in an adjacent one.
Perception	Perception is the process of acquiring, interpreting, selecting, and organizing sensory information.
Attention	Attention is the cognitive process of selectively concentrating on one thing while ignoring other things. Psychologists have labeled three types of attention: sustained attention, selective attention, and divided attention.
Visible spectrum	The narrow band of electromagnetic waves, 380-760 nm in length, that are visible to the human eye is referred to as the visible spectrum.
Reflection	Reflection is the process of rephrasing or repeating thoughts and feelings expressed, making the person more aware of what they are saying or thinking.
Hue	A hue refers to the gradation of color within the optical spectrum, or visible spectrum, of light. Hue may also refer to a particular color within this spectrum, as defined by its dominant wavelength, or the central tendency of its combined wavelengths.
Saturation	Saturation refers to the degree to which the light waves producing a color are of the same wavelength. It is the purity of a color.
Theories	Theories are logically self-consistent models or frameworks describing the behavior of a certain natural or social phenomenon. They are broad explanations and predictions concerning phenomena of interest.
Physiology	The study of the functions and activities of living cells, tissues, and organs and of the physical and chemical phenomena involved is referred to as physiology.
Neuron	The neuron is the primary cell of the nervous system. They are found in the brain, the spinal cord, in the nerves and ganglia of the peripheral nervous system. It is a specialized cell that conducts impulses through the nervous system and contains three major parts: cell body, dendrites, and an axon. It can have many dendrites but only one axon.
Trichromatic theory	The trichromatic theory was postulated by Young and later by Helmholtz. They demonstrated that most colors can be matched by superimposing three separate light sources known as primaries; a process known as additive mixing. The Young-Helmholtz theory of color vision was built around the assumption of there being three classes of receptors.
Thomas Young	Thomas Young discovered that light was composed of waves through his famous double-slit experiment and described the process of accomodation of vision as a result of the change of the curvature of the lens. He also argued that color perception depends on the presence in the retina of three kinds of nerve fibres which respond respectively to red, green and violet light.
Helmholtz	Helmholtz a pioneer of the new science of psychology, was a rigorous experimental physiologist and philospher. He gave us the distinction between sensation and peception and is well known for his theories of color perception and hearing.
Rods	Rods are cylindrical shaped photoreceptors that are sensitive to the intensity of light. Rods require less light to function than cone cells, and therefore are the primary source of visual information at night.

Go to **Cram101.com** for the Practice Tests for this Chapter.

Chapter 6. Perceiving Color

Chapter 6. Perceiving Color

Contrast effect	A contrast effect is the enhancement or diminishment, relative to normal, of a perception and related performance as a result of immediately previous or simultaneous exposure to a stimulus of lesser or greater value in the same dimension.
Adaptation	Adaptation is a lowering of sensitivity to a stimulus following prolonged exposure to that stimulus. Behavioral adaptations are special ways a particular organism behaves to survive in its natural habitat.
Nervous system	The body's electrochemical communication circuitry, made up of billions of neurons is a nervous system.
Amino acid	Amino acid is the basic structural building unit of proteins. They form short polymer chains called peptides or polypeptides which in turn form structures called proteins.
Cones	Cones are photoreceptors that transmit sensations of color, function in bright light, and used in visual acuity. Infants prior to months of age can only distinguish green and red indicating the cones are not fully developed; they can see all of the colors by 2 months of
Photon	A photon is a quantum of the electromagnetic field, for instance light. In some respects a photon acts as a particle, for instance when registered by the light sensitive device in a camera. It also acts like a wave, as when passing through the optics in a camera.
Opponent-process theory	The opponent-process theory is a color theory that states that the human visual system interprets information about color by processing signals from cones in an antagonistic manner.
Hering	Hering disagreed with the trichromatic theory of color perception which held that the human eye perceived all colors in terms of three primary colors. (Red, Green, Blue). He believed that the visual system worked based on a system of color opponency, a system of six primary colors.
Afterimage	An afterimage is an optical illusion that occurs after looking away from a direct gaze at an image. This is closely related to the phenomenon called the persistence of vision, which is used in animation and cinema.
Quantitative	A quantitative property is one that exists in a range of magnitudes, and can therefore be measured. Measurements of any particular quantitative property are expressed as as a specific quantity, referred to as a unit, multiplied by a number.
Sensation	Sensation is the first stage in the chain of biochemical and neurologic events that begins with the impinging of a stimulus upon the receptor cells of a sensory organ, which then leads to perception, the mental state that is reflected in statements like "I see a uniformly blue wall."
Stimulus	A change in an environmental condition that elicits a response is a stimulus.
Retina	The retina is a thin layer of cells at the back of the eyeball. It is the part of the eye which converts light into nervous signals. The retina contains photoreceptor cells which receive the light; the resulting neural signals then undergo complex processing by other neurons of the retina, and are transformed into action potentials in retinal ganglion cells whose axons form the optic nerve.
Lateral geniculate nucleus	The lateral geniculate nucleus of the thalamus is a part of the brain, which is the primary processor of visual information, received from the retina, in the CNS.
Nerve	A nerve is an enclosed, cable-like bundle of nerve fibers or axons, which includes the glia that ensheath the axons in myelin. Neurons are sometimes called nerve cells, though this term is technically imprecise since many neurons do not form nerves.

Go to **Cram101.com** for the Practice Tests for this Chapter.

Chapter 6. Perceiving Color

Bipolar cell	As a part of the retina, the bipolar cell exists between photoreceptors and ganglion cells. Bipolar cells are so-named as they have a central body from which two sets of processes arise. At one end, they form synapses with either a single cone cell, or a number of rod cells. At the other end, they form synapses with ganglion cells, which fire action potentials along the optic nerve (cranial nerve II). They effectively transfer information from rods and cones to ganglion cells.
Coding	In senation, coding is the process by which information about the quality and quantity of a stimulus is preserved in the pattern of action potentials sent through sensory neurons to the central nervous system.
Excitatory synapse	An excitatory synapse is where the neurotransmitter increases the likelihood that an action potential will occur, or increases the rate at which they are already occurring, in the neuron on which it acts.
Striate cortex	The functionally defined primary visual cortex is approximately equivalent to the anatomically defined striate cortex located in the occipital lobe.
Visual acuity	Visual acuity is the eye's ability to detect fine details and is the quantitative measure of the eye's ability to see an in-focus image at a certain distance.
Brain	The brain controls and coordinates most movement, behavior and homeostatic body functions such as heartbeat, blood pressure, fluid balance and body temperature. Functions of the brain are responsible for cognition, emotion, memory, motor learning and other sorts of learning. The brain is primarily made up of two types of cells: glia and neurons.
Trichromat	A trichromat is an organism for which the perceptual effect of any chosen light from its visible spectrum can be matched by a mixture of no more than three different pure spectral lights. The organism's retina contains three types of color receptors with different absorption spectra.
Dichromat	A person who is insensitive to the colors of red and green and hence partially color blind is called dichromat.
Monochromat	A monochromat is an organism that is truly color blind. That is, the perceptual effect of any arbitrarily chosen light from its visible spectrum can be matched by any pure spectral light. Monochromats can only see shades of black, gray and white.
Graham	Graham has conducted a number of studies that reveal stronger socioeconomic-status influences rather than ethnic influences in achievement.
X chromosome	The sex chromosomes are one of the 23 pairs of human chromosomes. Each person normally has one pair of sex chromosomes in each cell. Females have two X chromosomes, while males have one X and one Y chromosome. The X chromosome carries hundreds of genes but few, if any, of these have anything to do directly with sex determination.
Chromosome	The DNA which carries genetic information in biological cells is normally packaged in the form of one or more large macromolecules called a chromosome. Humans normally have 46.
Gene	A gene is an ultramicroscopic area of the chromosome. It is the smallest physical unit of the DNA molecule that carries a piece of hereditary information.
Affect	A subjective feeling or emotional tone often accompanied by bodily expressions noticeable to others is called affect.
Neural impulse	Neural impulse refers to the electrochemical discharge of a nerve cell, or neuron.
Color constancy	Color constancy is an example of subjective constancy and a feature of the human color-perception system which ensures that the perceived color of objects remains relatively constant under varying illumination conditions in spite of physical change.

Chapter 6. Perceiving Color

Chapter 6. Perceiving Color

Lightness constancy	Lightness constancy refers to the perceptual tendency to perceive a surface as having the same degree of lightness or darkness regardless of the amount of light that illuminates it.
Evolution	Commonly used to refer to gradual change, evolution is the change in the frequency of alleles within a population from one generation to the next. This change may be caused by different mechanisms, including natural selection, genetic drift, or changes in population (gene flow).
Fovea	The fovea, a part of the eye, is a spot located in the center of the macula. The fovea is responsible for sharp central vision, which is necessary in humans for reading, watching television or movies, driving, and any activity where visual detail is of primary importance.
Attitude	An enduring mental representation of a person, place, or thing that evokes an emotional response and related behavior is called attitude.
Plasticity	The capacity for modification and change is referred to as plasticity.
Senses	The senses are systems that consist of a sensory cell type that respond to a specific kind of physical energy, and that correspond to a defined region within the brain where the signals are received and interpreted.
Top-down	In the Top-down model an overview of the system is formulated, without going into detail for any part of it. Each part of the system is then refined by designing it in more detail. Each new part may then be refined again, defining it in yet more detail until the entire specification is detailed enough to validate the Model.

Chapter 6. Perceiving Color

Chapter 7. Perceiving Depth and Size

Retina	The retina is a thin layer of cells at the back of the eyeball. It is the part of the eye which converts light into nervous signals. The retina contains photoreceptor cells which receive the light; the resulting neural signals then undergo complex processing by other neurons of the retina, and are transformed into action potentials in retinal ganglion cells whose axons form the optic nerve.
Perception	Perception is the process of acquiring, interpreting, selecting, and organizing sensory information.
Depth cues	Perceptual features that impart information about distance and three-dimensional space are called depth cues.
Learning	Learning is a relatively permanent change in behavior that results from experience. Thus, to attribute a behavioral change to learning, the change must be relatively permanent and must result from experience.
Accommodation	Piaget's developmental process of accommodation is the modification of currently held schemes or new schemes so that new information inconsistent with the existing schemes can be integrated and understood.
Monocular	Depth perception combines several types of depth clues grouped into two categories: monocular clues, available from the input of just one eye, and binocular clues. Monocular clues include motion parallax, color vision, perspective, relative size, distance fog, depth from focus, and occlusion
Occlusion	The monocular depth cue occlusion is the blocking of sight of objects by other objects. It creates a "ranking" of nearness, and does not give any insight as to actual distances. In the absence of color or binocular vision, it often serves as the method of last resort for rudimentary depth perception.
Relative size	Relative size is a monocular cue where an an automobile that is close to us seems larger than one that is far away. The visual system exploits the relative size of similar (or familiar) objects to judge distance.
Illusion	An illusion is a distortion of a sensory perception.
Linear perspective	A monocular depth cue, linear perspective is the property of parallel lines converging at infinity allowing us to reconstruct the relative distance of two parts of an object, or of landscape features.
Texture gradient	Texture gradient is a monocular cue for depth based on the perception that closer objects appear to have rougher surfaces. Objects appear denser as they go further away.
Motion parallax	A monocular cue for depth, motion parallax is the apparent relative motion of several stationary objects against a background when the observer moves gives hints about their relative distance. This effect can be seen clearly when driving in a car, nearby things pass quickly, while far off objects appear stationary.
Helmholtz	Helmholtz a pioneer of the new science of psychology, was a rigorous experimental physiologist and philospher. He gave us the distinction between sensation and peception and is well known for his theories of color perception and hearing.
Binocular depth cues	Binocular depth cues that depend on two eyes working together.
Binocular cue	A stimulus suggestive of depth that involves simultaneous perception by both eyes is a binocular cue. Convergence is a binocular cue for depth based on the inward movement of the eyes as they attempt to focus on an object that is drawing nearer.
Binocular	A binocular depth cue resulting from differences between the two retinal images formed of an

Chapter 7. Perceiving Depth and Size

Chapter 7. Perceiving Depth and Size

disparity	object viewed at distances up to about 20 feet is referred to as binocular disparity.
Stereopsis	Stereopsis is the process in visual perception leading to perception of the depth or distance of objects. Depth from stereopsis arises from the slightly different positions each eye occupies on the head, a form of parallax.
Stages	Stages represent relatively discrete periods of time in which functioning is qualitatively different from functioning at other periods.
Polarization	Polarization is the process of preparing a neuron for firing by creating an internal negative charge in relation to the body fluid outside the cell membrane.
Visual cortex	The visual cortex is the general term applied to both the primary visual cortex and the visual association area. Anatomically, the visual cortex occupies the entire occipital lobe, the inferior temporal lobe (IT), posterior parts of the parietal lobe, and a few small regions in the frontal lobe.
Fovea	The fovea, a part of the eye, is a spot located in the center of the macula. The fovea is responsible for sharp central vision, which is necessary in humans for reading, watching television or movies, driving, and any activity where visual detail is of primary importance.
Fixation	Fixation in abnormal psychology is the state where an individual becomes obsessed with an attachment to another human, animal or inanimate object. Fixation in vision refers to maintaining the gaze in a constant direction. .
Pictorial cues	Pictorial cues for depth perception operate on real scenes and when viewing pictures. They include occlusion, relative image size for familiar objects, linear perspective, texture gradient, differential lighting of surfaces, and position relative location.
Stimulus	A change in an environmental condition that elicits a response is a stimulus.
Retinal disparity	A binocular cue for depth based on the difference in the image cast by an object on the retinas of the eyes as the object moves closer or farther away, is called retinal disparity.
Neuron	The neuron is the primary cell of the nervous system. They are found in the brain, the spinal cord, in the nerves and ganglia of the peripheral nervous system. It is a specialized cell that conducts impulses through the nervous system and contains three major parts: cell body, dendrites, and an axon. It can have many dendrites but only one axon.
Histogram	In statistics, a histogram is a graphical display of tabulated frequencies. It is the graphical version of a table which shows what proportion of cases fall into each of several or many specified categories. The categories are usually specified as nonoverlapping intervals of some variable.
Brain	The brain controls and coordinates most movement, behavior and homeostatic body functions such as heartbeat, blood pressure, fluid balance and body temperature. Functions of the brain are responsible for cognition, emotion, memory, motor learning and other sorts of learning. The brain is primarily made up of two types of cells: glia and neurons.
Survey	A method of scientific investigation in which a large sample of people answer questions about their attitudes or behavior is referred to as a survey.
Anatomy	Anatomy is the branch of biology that deals with the structure and organization of living things. It can be divided into animal anatomy (zootomy) and plant anatomy (phytonomy). Major branches of anatomy include comparative anatomy, histology, and human anatomy.
Physiology	The study of the functions and activities of living cells, tissues, and organs and of the physical and chemical phenomena involved is referred to as physiology.
Brain imaging	Brain imaging is a fairly recent discipline within medicine and neuroscience. Brain imaging falls into two broad categories -- structural imaging and functional imaging.

Go to Cram101.com for the Practice Tests for this Chapter.

Chapter 7. Perceiving Depth and Size

Chapter 7. Perceiving Depth and Size

Species	Species refers to a reproductively isolated breeding population.
Parallax	Parallax is the apparent shift of an object against a background due to a change in observer position.
Edwin Boring	Edwin Boring is one of the first historians of psychology.
Size constancy	The tendency to perceive an object as being the same size even as the size of its retinal image changes according to the object's distance is referred to as size constancy.
Afterimage	An afterimage is an optical illusion that occurs after looking away from a direct gaze at an image. This is closely related to the phenomenon called the persistence of vision, which is used in animation and cinema.
Visual illusion	Visual illusion refers to a discrepancy or incongruency between reality and the perceptual representation of it.
Variable	A variable refers to a measurable factor, characteristic, or attribute of an individual or a system.
Ponzo	The Ponzo Illusion illustrates that the human mind judges an objects size based on its background. Two identical lines are drawn across a pair of converging lines, similar to railway tracks. The upper bar looked wider because it spans a greater apparent distance between the rails.
Ames room	An Ames room is a distorted room that is used to create an optical illusion. As a result of the optical illusion, a person standing in one corner appears to the observer to be a giant while a person standing in the other corner appears to be a midget.
Moon illusion	The moon illusion is an optical illusion in which the moon appears larger near the horizon than it does while higher up in the sky. This optical illusion also occurs with the sun and star constellations.
Sensitive period	A sensitive period is a developmental window in which a predisposed behavior is most likely to develop given appropriate stimulation. In linguistic theory, the period from about 18 months to puberty is when the brain is thought to be primed for learning language because of plasticity of the brain.
Binocular vision	Binocular vision is vision in which both eyes are used synchronously to produce a single image. It confers two advantages over monocular vision: binocular summation in which the ability to detect faint objects is enhanced, and stereopsis in which parallax provided by the two eye's different positions on the head give precise depth perception.
Visual acuity	Visual acuity is the eye's ability to detect fine details and is the quantitative measure of the eye's ability to see an in-focus image at a certain distance.
Attention	Attention is the cognitive process of selectively concentrating on one thing while ignoring other things. Psychologists have labeled three types of attention: sustained attention, selective attention, and divided attention.
Plasticity	The capacity for modification and change is referred to as plasticity.
Deprivation	Deprivation, is the loss or withholding of normal stimulation, nutrition, comfort, love, and so forth; a condition of lacking. The level of stimulation is less than what is required.
Senses	The senses are systems that consist of a sensory cell type that respond to a specific kind of physical energy, and that correspond to a defined region within the brain where the signals are received and interpreted.

Go to Cram101.com for the Practice Tests for this Chapter.

Chapter 7. Perceiving Depth and Size

Chapter 8. Perceiving Movement

Retina	The retina is a thin layer of cells at the back of the eyeball. It is the part of the eye which converts light into nervous signals. The retina contains photoreceptor cells which receive the light; the resulting neural signals then undergo complex processing by other neurons of the retina, and are transformed into action potentials in retinal ganglion cells whose axons form the optic nerve.
Perception	Perception is the process of acquiring, interpreting, selecting, and organizing sensory information.
Motion perception	Motion perception is the process of inferring the "true" velocity and direction of motion in a visual scene given some visual input.
Nervous system	The body's electrochemical communication circuitry, made up of billions of neurons is a nervous system.
Stimulus	A change in an environmental condition that elicits a response is a stimulus.
Heuristic	A heuristic is a simple, efficient rule of thumb proposed to explain how people make decisions, come to judgments and solve problems, typically when facing complex problems or incomplete information. These rules work well under most circumstances, but in certain cases lead to systematic cognitive biases.
Top-down	In the Top-down model an overview of the system is formulated, without going into detail for any part of it. Each part of the system is then refined by designing it in more detail. Each new part may then be refined again, defining it in yet more detail until the entire specification is detailed enough to validate the Model.
Threshold	In general, a threshold is a fixed location or value where an abrupt change is observed. In the sensory modalities, it is the minimum amount of stimulus energy necessary to elicit a sensory response.
Affect	A subjective feeling or emotional tone often accompanied by bodily expressions noticeable to others is called affect.
Apparent movement	Apparent movement is the perceived motion of an object when all that has been presented to the eyes is one or a series of stills.
Gestalt psychology	According to Gestalt psychology, people naturally organize their perceptions according to certain patterns. The tendency is to organize perceptions into wholes and to integrate separate stimuli into meaningful patterns.
Wertheimer	His discovery of the phi phenomenon concerning the illusion of motion gave rise to the influential school of Gestalt psychology. In the latter part of his life, Wertheimer directed much of his attention to the problem of learning.
Illusion	An illusion is a distortion of a sensory perception.
Stages	Stages represent relatively discrete periods of time in which functioning is qualitatively different from functioning at other periods.
Feature detector	A feature detector is sensory system that is highly attuned to a specific stimulus pattern. They are nerve cells in the brain that respond to specific features of the stimulus, such as shape, angle, or movement.
Hubel and Weisel	Hubel and Weisel advanced the theory that receptive fields of cells at one level of the visual system are formed from input by cells at a lower level of the visual system.
Neuron	The neuron is the primary cell of the nervous system. They are found in the brain, the spinal cord, in the nerves and ganglia of the peripheral nervous system. It is a specialized cell that conducts impulses through the nervous system and contains three major parts: cell body, dendrites, and an axon. It can have many dendrites but only one axon.

Chapter 8. Perceiving Movement

Chapter 8. Perceiving Movement

Receptor	A sensory receptor is a structure that recognizes a stimulus in the internal or external environment of an organism. In response to stimuli the sensory receptor initiates sensory transduction by creating graded potentials or action potentials in the same cell or in an adjacent one.
Dorsal stream	The dorsal stream is a pathway for visual information which flows through the visual cortex, the part of the brain which provides visual processing. It is involved in spatial awareness: recognizing where objects are in space.
Receptive field	The receptive field of a sensory neuron is a region of sensitivity in which the presence of a stimulus will alter the firing of that neuron.
Visual cortex	The visual cortex is the general term applied to both the primary visual cortex and the visual association area. Anatomically, the visual cortex occupies the entire occipital lobe, the inferior temporal lobe (IT), posterior parts of the parietal lobe, and a few small regions in the frontal lobe.
Afterimage	An afterimage is an optical illusion that occurs after looking away from a direct gaze at an image. This is closely related to the phenomenon called the persistence of vision, which is used in animation and cinema.
Synchrony	In child development, synchrony is the carefully coordinated interaction between the parent and the child or adolescent in which, often unknowingly, they are attuned to each other's behavior.
Fovea	The fovea, a part of the eye, is a spot located in the center of the macula. The fovea is responsible for sharp central vision, which is necessary in humans for reading, watching television or movies, driving, and any activity where visual detail is of primary importance.
Fixation	Fixation in abnormal psychology is the state where an individual becomes obsessed with an attachment to another human, animal or inanimate object. Fixation in vision refers to maintaining the gaze in a constant direction. .
Agnosia	Agnosia is a loss of ability to recognize objects, persons, sounds, shapes or smells while the specific sense is not defective nor is there any significant memory loss. It is usually associated with brain injury or neurological illness, particularly after damage to the temporal lobe.
Striate cortex	The functionally defined primary visual cortex is approximately equivalent to the anatomically defined striate cortex located in the occipital lobe.
Law of common fate	The Gestalt Law of Common Fate argues that elements having the apparent same moving direction are seen as a unit.
Brain	The brain controls and coordinates most movement, behavior and homeostatic body functions such as heartbeat, blood pressure, fluid balance and body temperature. Functions of the brain are responsible for cognition, emotion, memory, motor learning and other sorts of learning. The brain is primarily made up of two types of cells: glia and neurons.
Occlusion	The monocular depth cue occlusion is the blocking of sight of objects by other objects. It creates a "ranking" of nearness, and does not give any insight as to actual distances. In the absence of color or binocular vision, it often serves as the method of last resort for rudimentary depth perception.
Apparent motion	Apparent motion is the perceived motion of an object when all that has been presented to the eyes is one or a series of stills.
Motor cortex	Motor cortex refers to the section of cortex that lies in the frontal lobe, just across the central fissure from the sensory cortex. Neural impulses in the motor cortex are linked to muscular responses throughout the body.

Chapter 8. Perceiving Movement

Chapter 8. Perceiving Movement

Tactile	Pertaining to the sense of touch is referred to as tactile.
Somatosensory	Somatosensory system consists of the various sensory receptors that trigger the experiences labelled as touch or pressure, temperature, pain, and the sensations of muscle movement and joint position including posture, movement, and facial expression.
Somatosensory cortex	The primary somatosensory cortex is across the central sulcus and behind the primary motor cortex configured to generally correspond with the arrangement of nearby motor cells related to specific body parts. It is the main sensory receptive area for the sense of touch.
Plasticity	The capacity for modification and change is referred to as plasticity.
Senses	The senses are systems that consist of a sensory cell type that respond to a specific kind of physical energy, and that correspond to a defined region within the brain where the signals are received and interpreted.

Chapter 8. Perceiving Movement

Chapter 9. Perception and Action

Perception	Perception is the process of acquiring, interpreting, selecting, and organizing sensory information.
Retina	The retina is a thin layer of cells at the back of the eyeball. It is the part of the eye which converts light into nervous signals. The retina contains photoreceptor cells which receive the light; the resulting neural signals then undergo complex processing by other neurons of the retina, and are transformed into action potentials in retinal ganglion cells whose axons form the optic nerve.
Size constancy	The tendency to perceive an object as being the same size even as the size of its retinal image changes according to the object's distance is referred to as size constancy.
Texture gradient	Texture gradient is a monocular cue for depth based on the perception that closer objects appear to have rougher surfaces. Objects appear denser as they go further away.
Invariance	Invariance is the property of perception whereby simple geometrical objects are recognized independent of rotation, translation, and scale, as well as several other variations such as elastic deformations, different lighting, and different component features.
Aronson	Aronson is credited with refining the theory of cognitive dissonance, which posits that when attitudes and behaviors are inconsistent with one another that psychological discomfort results. This discomfort motivates the person experiencing it to either change their behavior or attitude so that consonance is restored.
Vestibular system	The vestibular system, or balance system, is the sensory system that provides the dominant input about our movement and orientation in space. Together with the cochlea, the auditory organ, it is situated in the vestibulum in the inner ear.
Inner ear	The inner ear consists of the oval window, cochlea, and basilar membrane.
Receptor	A sensory receptor is a structure that recognizes a stimulus in the internal or external environment of an organism. In response to stimuli the sensory receptor initiates sensory transduction by creating graded potentials or action potentials in the same cell or in an adjacent one.
Toddler	A toddler is a child between the ages of one and three years old. During this period, the child learns a great deal about social roles and develops motor skills; to toddle is to walk unsteadily.
Variable	A variable refers to a measurable factor, characteristic, or attribute of an individual or a system.
Binocular vision	Binocular vision is vision in which both eyes are used synchronously to produce a single image. It confers two advantages over monocular vision: binocular summation in which the ability to detect faint objects is enhanced, and stereopsis in which parallax provided by the two eye's different positions on the head give precise depth perception.
Affect	A subjective feeling or emotional tone often accompanied by bodily expressions noticeable to others is called affect.
Neuron	The neuron is the primary cell of the nervous system. They are found in the brain, the spinal cord, in the nerves and ganglia of the peripheral nervous system. It is a specialized cell that conducts impulses through the nervous system and contains three major parts: cell body, dendrites, and an axon. It can have many dendrites but only one axon.
Nucleus	In neuroanatomy, a cluster of cell bodies of neurons within the central nervous system is a nucleus.
Brain	The brain controls and coordinates most movement, behavior and homeostatic body functions such as heartbeat, blood pressure, fluid balance and body temperature. Functions of the brain

Chapter 9. Perception and Action

Chapter 9. Perception and Action

	are responsible for cognition, emotion, memory, motor learning and other sorts of learning. The brain is primarily made up of two types of cells: glia and neurons.
Dorsal stream	The dorsal stream is a pathway for visual information which flows through the visual cortex, the part of the brain which provides visual processing. It is involved in spatial awareness: recognizing where objects are in space.
Receptive field	The receptive field of a sensory neuron is a region of sensitivity in which the presence of a stimulus will alter the firing of that neuron.
Stimulus	A change in an environmental condition that elicits a response is a stimulus.
Visual perception	Visual perception is one of the senses, consisting of the ability to detect light and interpret it. Vision has a specific sensory system.
Extrastriate cortex	The extrastriate cortex is the locus of mid-level vision. Neurons in the extrastriate cortex generally respond to visual stimuli within their receptive fields. These responses are modulated by extraretinal effects, like attention, working memory, and reward expectation.
Frontal lobe	The frontal lobe comprises four major folds of cortical tissue: the precentral gyrus, superior gyrus and the middle gyrus of the frontal gyri, the inferior frontal gyrus. It has been found to play a part in impulse control, judgement, language, memory, motor function, problem solving, sexual behavior, socialization and spontaneity.
Motor cortex	Motor cortex refers to the section of cortex that lies in the frontal lobe, just across the central fissure from the sensory cortex. Neural impulses in the motor cortex are linked to muscular responses throughout the body.
Parietal lobe	The parietal lobe is positioned above (superior to) the occipital lobe and behind (posterior to) the frontal lobe. It plays important roles in integrating sensory information from various senses, and in the manipulation of objects.
Motor neuron	A motor neuron is an efferent neuron that originates in the spinal cord and synapses with muscle fibers to facilitate muscle contraction and with muscle spindles to modify proprioceptive sensitivity.
Senses	The senses are systems that consist of a sensory cell type that respond to a specific kind of physical energy, and that correspond to a defined region within the brain where the signals are received and interpreted.

Chapter 10. Sound, the Auditory System and Pitch Perception

Stimulus	A change in an environmental condition that elicits a response is a stimulus.
Auditory system	The auditory system is the sensory system for the sense of hearing. On its path from the outside world to the forebrain, sound information is preserved and modified in many ways. It changes media twice, first from air to fluid, then from fluid to action potentials.
Perception	Perception is the process of acquiring, interpreting, selecting, and organizing sensory information.
Pitch	Pitch is the psychological interpretation of a sound or musical tone corresponding to its physical frequency
Affect	A subjective feeling or emotional tone often accompanied by bodily expressions noticeable to others is called affect.
Amplitude	Amplitude is a nonnegative scalar measure of a wave's magnitude of oscillation.
Loudness	Loudness is the quality of a sound that is the primary psychological correlate of physical intensity. Loudness is often approximated by a power function with an exponent of 0.6 when plotted vs. sound pressure or 0.3 when plotted vs. sound intensity.
Graham	Graham has conducted a number of studies that reveal stronger socioeconomic-status influences rather than ethnic influences in achievement.
Fundamental frequency	The fundamental frequency of a periodic signal is the inverse of the pitch period length. The pitch period is, in turn, the smallest repeating unit of a signal.
Visible spectrum	The narrow band of electromagnetic waves, 380-760 nm in length, that are visible to the human eye is referred to as the visible spectrum.
Threshold	In general, a threshold is a fixed location or value where an abrupt change is observed. In the sensory modalities, it is the minimum amount of stimulus energy necessary to elicit a sensory response.
Sensation	Sensation is the first stage in the chain of biochemical and neurologic events that begins with the impinging of a stimulus upon the receptor cells of a sensory organ, which then leads to perception, the mental state that is reflected in statements like "I see a uniformly blue wall."
Cochlea	The Cochlea is the bony tube that contains the basilar membrane and the organ of Corti. The cochlea consists of three fluid-filled chambers - scala tympani and scala vestibuli and scala media.
Timbre	The distinctive quality of a sound that distinguishes it from other sounds of the same pitch and loudness is called timbre.
Outer ear	Outer ear consists of the pinna and the external auditory canal.
Middle ear	The middle ear consists of the eardrum, hammer, anvil, and stirrup.
Pinna	The pinna is the visible part of the ear that resides outside of the head. It acts as a funnel, amplifying the sound and directing it to the ear canal. While reflecting from the pinna, sound also goes through a filtering process which adds directional information to the sound.
Tympanic membrane	The tympanic membrane, colloquially known as eardrum, is a thin membrane that separates the outer ear from the middle ear. Its function is to transmit sound from the air to the ossicles inside the middle ear.
Eardrum	The tympanum or tympanic membrane, colloquially known as the eardrum, is a thin membrane that separates the outer ear from the middle ear. Its function is to transmit sound from the air to the ossicles inside the middle ear. The malleus bone connects the eardrum to the other

Chapter 10. Sound, the Auditory System and Pitch Perception

Chapter 10. Sound, the Auditory System and Pitch Perception

	ossicles.
Auditory nerve	The vestibulocochlear nerve is the eighth of twelve cranial nerves, and also known as the auditory nerve. It is the nerve along which the sensory cells (the hair cells) of the inner ear transmit information to the brain. It consists of the cochlear nerve, carrying information about hearing, and the vestibular nerve, carrying information about balance.
Oval window	The oval window is a membrane-covered opening which leads from the middle ear to the vestibule of the inner ear.
Malleus	The malleus is hammer-shaped small bone or ossicle of the middle ear which connects with the incus and is attached to the inner surface of the eardrum.
Stapes	The stapes or stirrup is the stirrup-shaped small bone or ossicle in the middle ear which attaches the incus to the fenestra ovalis, the "oval window" which is adjacent to the vestibule of the inner ear. It is the smallest bone in the human body.
Inner ear	The inner ear consists of the oval window, cochlea, and basilar membrane.
Ossicles	The ossicles are the three smallest bones in the human body. They are contained within the middle ear space and serve to transmit sounds from the air to the fluid filled labyrinth (cochlea).
Skeletal muscle	Skeletal muscle is a type of striated muscle, attached to the skeleton. They are used to facilitate movement, by applying force to bones and joints; via contraction. They generally contract voluntarily (via nerve stimulation), although they can contract involuntarily.
Organ of Corti	The Organ of Corti is the hearing organ of the inner ear. It contains receptors that respond to vibrations in the basilar membrane which are caused by sound.
Basilar membrane	The basilar membrane within the cochlea of the inner ear is the part of the auditory system that decomposes incoming auditory signals into their frequency components. This allows higher neural processing of sound information to focus on the frequency spectrum of input, rather than just the time domain waveform.
Hair cells	Hair cells are the sensory cells of both the auditory system and the vestibular system. The auditory hair cells are located within the organ of Corti on a thin basilar membrane in the cochlea of the inner ear.
Receptor	A sensory receptor is a structure that recognizes a stimulus in the internal or external environment of an organism. In response to stimuli the sensory receptor initiates sensory transduction by creating graded potentials or action potentials in the same cell or in an adjacent one.
Transducer	A device that converts energy from one system into energy in another is referred to as transducer.
Neurotransmitter	A neurotransmitter is a chemical that is used to relay, amplify and modulate electrical signals between a neurons and another cell.
Nerve	A nerve is an enclosed, cable-like bundle of nerve fibers or axons, which includes the glia that ensheath the axons in myelin. Neurons are sometimes called nerve cells, though this term is technically imprecise since many neurons do not form nerves.
Brain	The brain controls and coordinates most movement, behavior and homeostatic body functions such as heartbeat, blood pressure, fluid balance and body temperature. Functions of the brain are responsible for cognition, emotion, memory, motor learning and other sorts of learning. The brain is primarily made up of two types of cells: glia and neurons.
Nucleus	In neuroanatomy, a cluster of cell bodies of neurons within the central nervous system is a nucleus.

Chapter 10. Sound, the Auditory System and Pitch Perception

Chapter 10. Sound, the Auditory System and Pitch Perception

Synapse	A synapse is specialized junction through which cells of the nervous system signal to one another and to non-neuronal cells such as muscles or glands.
Brain stem	The brain stem is the stalk of the brain below the cerebral hemispheres. It is the major route for communication between the forebrain and the spinal cord and peripheral nerves. It also controls various functions including respiration, regulation of heart rhythms, and primary aspects of sound localization.
Midbrain	Located between the hindbrain and forebrain, a region in which many nerve-fiber systems ascend and descend to connect the higher and lower portions of the brain is referred to as midbrain. It is archipallian in origin, meaning its general architecture is shared with the most ancient of vertebrates. Dopamine produced in the subtantia nigra plays a role in motivation and habituation of species from humans to the most elementary animals such as insects.
Thalamus	An area near the center of the brain involved in the relay of sensory information to the cortex and in the functions of sleep and attention is the thalamus.
Traveling wave	The pattern of vibration in the cochlear fluid, which varies as a function of the amplitude and frequency of an airborne sound is referred to as a traveling wave.
Displacement	An unconscious defense mechanism in which the individual directs aggressive or sexual feelings away from the primary object to someone or something safe is referred to as displacement. Displacement in linguistics is simply the ability to talk about things not present.
Coding	In senation, coding is the process by which information about the quality and quantity of a stimulus is preserved in the pattern of action potentials sent through sensory neurons to the central nervous system.
Electrode	Any device used to electrically stimulate nerve tissue or to record its activity is an electrode.
Microelectrode	An electrical wire so small that it can be used either to monitor the electrical activity of a single neuron or to stimulate activity within it is a microelectrode.
Auditory masking	The phenomenon by which one sound tends to prevent the hearing of another sound is called auditory masking.
Place theory	Place theory is a theory of hearing which states that our perception of sound depends on where each component frequency produces vibrations along the basilar membrane. It was first discovered by Helmholtz.
Nerve impulse	A nerve impulse is a change in the electric potential of a neuron; a wave of depolarization spreads along the neuron and causes the release of a neurotransmitter.
Analyzer	Pavlov's name for a specialized part of the nervous system is Analyzer, which controls the reactions of the organism to changing external conditions. It consists of sense rescептors, the sensory pathway to the cortex, and the area of the cortex where the sensory activity is projected.
Temporal lobe	The temporal lobe is part of the cerebrum. It lies at the side of the brain, beneath the lateral or Sylvian fissure. Adjacent areas in the superior, posterior and lateral parts of the temporal lobe are involved in high-level auditory processing.
Primary auditory cortex	The primary auditory cortex is responsible for processing of auditory information. It is located in the temporal lobe; the posterior half of the superior temporal gyrus and also dives into the lateral sulcus as the transverse temporal gyri.
Association	Association areas refer to the site of the higher mental processes such as thought, language,

Chapter 10. Sound, the Auditory System and Pitch Perception

Chapter 10. Sound, the Auditory System and Pitch Perception

areas	memory, and speech.
Frontal lobe	The frontal lobe comprises four major folds of cortical tissue: the precentral gyrus, superior gyrus and the middle gyrus of the frontal gyri, the inferior frontal gyrus. It has been found to play a part in impulse control, judgement, language, memory, motor function, problem solving, sexual behavior, socialization and spontaneity.
Neuron	The neuron is the primary cell of the nervous system. They are found in the brain, the spinal cord, in the nerves and ganglia of the peripheral nervous system. It is a specialized cell that conducts impulses through the nervous system and contains three major parts: cell body, dendrites, and an axon. It can have many dendrites but only one axon.
Plasticity	The capacity for modification and change is referred to as plasticity.
Brain imaging	Brain imaging is a fairly recent discipline within medicine and neuroscience. Brain imaging falls into two broad categories -- structural imaging and functional imaging.
Brightness	The dimension of visual sensation that is dependent on the intensity of light reflected from a surface and that corresponds to the amplitude of the light wave is called brightness.
Senses	The senses are systems that consist of a sensory cell type that respond to a specific kind of physical energy, and that correspond to a defined region within the brain where the signals are received and interpreted.
Association cortex	Region of the cerebral cortex in which the highest intellectual functions, including thinking and problem solving, occur is the association cortex.

Go to **Cram101.com** for the Practice Tests for this Chapter.

Chapter 10. Sound, the Auditory System and Pitch Perception

Chapter 11. Auditory Localization, Sound Quality and the Auditory Scene

Auditory localization	The perceptual ability to locate the source of a sound is called auditory localization. There are two general methods, binaural cues and monaural cues.
Sound localization	Sound localization is a listener's ability to identify the location of origin of a detected sound. There are two general methods for sound localization, binaural cues and monaural cues.
Variability	Statistically, variability refers to how much the scores in a distribution spread out, away from the mean.
Auditory system	The auditory system is the sensory system for the sense of hearing. On its path from the outside world to the forebrain, sound information is preserved and modified in many ways. It changes media twice, first from air to fluid, then from fluid to action potentials.
Retina	The retina is a thin layer of cells at the back of the eyeball. It is the part of the eye which converts light into nervous signals. The retina contains photoreceptor cells which receive the light; the resulting neural signals then undergo complex processing by other neurons of the retina, and are transformed into action potentials in retinal ganglion cells whose axons form the optic nerve.
Cochlea	The Cochlea is the bony tube that contains the basilar membrane and the organ of Corti. The cochlea consists of three fluid-filled chambers - scala tympani and scala vestibuli and scala media.
Binaural cue	A binaural cue relies on the comparison of auditory input from two separate detectors. The primary biological binaural cue is the split-second delay between the time when sound from a single source reaches the near ear and when it reaches the far ear.
Prototype	A concept of a category of objects or events that serves as a good example of the category is called a prototype.
Stimulus	A change in an environmental condition that elicits a response is a stimulus.
Affect	A subjective feeling or emotional tone often accompanied by bodily expressions noticeable to others is called affect.
Attention	Attention is the cognitive process of selectively concentrating on one thing while ignoring other things. Psychologists have labeled three types of attention: sustained attention, selective attention, and divided attention.
Parallax	Parallax is the apparent shift of an object against a background due to a change in observer position.
Reflection	Reflection is the process of rephrasing or repeating thoughts and feelings expressed, making the person more aware of what they are saying or thinking.
Perception	Perception is the process of acquiring, interpreting, selecting, and organizing sensory information.
Threshold	In general, a threshold is a fixed location or value where an abrupt change is observed. In the sensory modalities, it is the minimum amount of stimulus energy necessary to elicit a sensory response.
Neuron	The neuron is the primary cell of the nervous system. They are found in the brain, the spinal cord, in the nerves and ganglia of the peripheral nervous system. It is a specialized cell that conducts impulses through the nervous system and contains three major parts: cell body, dendrites, and an axon. It can have many dendrites but only one axon.
Nucleus	In neuroanatomy, a cluster of cell bodies of neurons within the central nervous system is a nucleus.
Right hemisphere	The brain is divided into left and right cerebral hemispheres. The right hemisphere of the

Go to Cram101.com for the Practice Tests for this Chapter.

Chapter 11. Auditory Localization, Sound Quality and the Auditory Scene

Chapter 11. Auditory Localization, Sound Quality and the Auditory Scene

	cortex controls the left side of the body.
Left hemisphere	The left hemisphere of the cortex controls the right side of the body, coordinates complex movements, and, in 95% of people, controls the production of speech and written language.
Primary auditory cortex	The primary auditory cortex is responsible for processing of auditory information. It is located in the temporal lobe; the posterior half of the superior temporal gyrus and also dives into the lateral sulcus as the transverse temporal gyri.
Nerve	A nerve is an enclosed, cable-like bundle of nerve fibers or axons, which includes the glia that ensheath the axons in myelin. Neurons are sometimes called nerve cells, though this term is technically imprecise since many neurons do not form nerves.
Senses	The senses are systems that consist of a sensory cell type that respond to a specific kind of physical energy, and that correspond to a defined region within the brain where the signals are received and interpreted.
Receptive field	The receptive field of a sensory neuron is a region of sensitivity in which the presence of a stimulus will alter the firing of that neuron.
Brain	The brain controls and coordinates most movement, behavior and homeostatic body functions such as heartbeat, blood pressure, fluid balance and body temperature. Functions of the brain are responsible for cognition, emotion, memory, motor learning and other sorts of learning. The brain is primarily made up of two types of cells: glia and neurons.
Pitch	Pitch is the psychological interpretation of a sound or musical tone corresponding to its physical frequency
Timbre	The distinctive quality of a sound that distinguishes it from other sounds of the same pitch and loudness is called timbre.
Fundamental frequency	The fundamental frequency of a periodic signal is the inverse of the pitch period length. The pitch period is, in turn, the smallest repeating unit of a signal.
Receptor	A sensory receptor is a structure that recognizes a stimulus in the internal or external environment of an organism. In response to stimuli the sensory receptor initiates sensory transduction by creating graded potentials or action potentials in the same cell or in an adjacent one.
Schema	Schema refers to a way of mentally representing the world, such as a belief or an expectation, that can influence perception of persons, objects, and situations.
Control group	A group that does not receive the treatment effect in an experiment is referred to as the control group or sometimes as the comparison group.
Somatosensory	Somatosensory system consists of the various sensory receptors that trigger the experiences labelled as touch or pressure, temperature, pain, and the sensations of muscle movement and joint position including posture, movement, and facial expression.
Deprivation	Deprivation, is the loss or withholding of normal stimulation, nutrition, comfort, love, and so forth; a condition of lacking. The level of stimulation is less than what is required.
Sulcus	A sulcus is a depression or fissure in the surface of an organ, most especially the brain. In the brain it surrounds the gyri, creating the characteristic appearance of the brain.
Plasticity	The capacity for modification and change is referred to as plasticity.

Chapter 11. Auditory Localization, Sound Quality and the Auditory Scene

Chapter 12. Speech Perception

Perception	Perception is the process of acquiring, interpreting, selecting, and organizing sensory information.
Plasticity	The capacity for modification and change is referred to as plasticity.
Nasal cavity	The nasal cavity is a large air-filled space above and behind the nose in the middle of the face. The nasal cavity is important in warming and cleaning the air as it is inhaled. The nasal cavity also contains organs involved in olfaction.
Larynx	The larynx, or voicebox, is an organ in the neck of mammals involved in protection of the trachea and sound production. The larynx houses the vocal cords, and is situated at the point where the upper tract splits into the trachea and the esophagus.
Stimulus	A change in an environmental condition that elicits a response is a stimulus.
Phoneme	In oral language, a phoneme is the theoretical basic unit of sound that can be used to distinguish words or morphemes; in sign language, it is a similarly basic unit of hand shape, motion, position, or facial expression.
Lungs	The lungs are the essential organs of respiration. Its principal function is to transport oxygen from the atmosphere into the bloodstream, and excrete carbon dioxide from the bloodstream into the atmosphere.
Amplitude	Amplitude is a nonnegative scalar measure of a wave's magnitude of oscillation.
Auditory system	The auditory system is the sensory system for the sense of hearing. On its path from the outside world to the forebrain, sound information is preserved and modified in many ways. It changes media twice, first from air to fluid, then from fluid to action potentials.
Variability	Statistically, variability refers to how much the scores in a distribution spread out, away from the mean.
Variable	A variable refers to a measurable factor, characteristic, or attribute of an individual or a system.
Perceptual constancy	Perceptual constancy is the recognition that objects are constant and unchanging even though sensory input about them is changing.
Invariance	Invariance is the property of perception whereby simple geometrical objects are recognized independent of rotation, translation, and scale, as well as several other variations such as elastic deformations, different lighting, and different component features.
Discrimination	In Learning theory, discrimination refers the ability to distinguish between a conditioned stimulus and other stimuli. It can be brought about by extensive training or differential reinforcement. In social terms, it is the denial of privileges to a person or a group on the basis of prejudice.
Visual cortex	The visual cortex is the general term applied to both the primary visual cortex and the visual association area. Anatomically, the visual cortex occupies the entire occipital lobe, the inferior temporal lobe (IT), posterior parts of the parietal lobe, and a few small regions in the frontal lobe.
Brain	The brain controls and coordinates most movement, behavior and homeostatic body functions such as heartbeat, blood pressure, fluid balance and body temperature. Functions of the brain are responsible for cognition, emotion, memory, motor learning and other sorts of learning. The brain is primarily made up of two types of cells: glia and neurons.
Senses	The senses are systems that consist of a sensory cell type that respond to a specific kind of physical energy, and that correspond to a defined region within the brain where the signals are received and interpreted.

Chapter 12. Speech Perception

Chapter 12. Speech Perception

Bottom-up processing	Using the parts of a pattern to recognize, or form an image of, the originating pattern is called bottom-up processing.
Top-down	In the Top-down model an overview of the system is formulated, without going into detail for any part of it. Each part of the system is then refined by designing it in more detail. Each new part may then be refined again, defining it in yet more detail until the entire specification is detailed enough to validate the Model.
Decoding	Process of phonetic analysis by which a printed word is converted to spoken form before retrieval from long-term memory is called decoding.
George Miller	George Miller provided two theoretical ideas that are fundamental to the information processing framework and cognitive psychology: chunking and the capacity of short term memory.
Long-term memory	Long-term memory is memory that lasts from over 30 seconds to years.
Control group	A group that does not receive the treatment effect in an experiment is referred to as the control group or sometimes as the comparison group.
Bottom-up	In Bottom-up design individual parts of the system are specified in detail. The parts are then linked together to form larger components, which are in turn linked until a complete system is formed. Strategies based on the bottom-up information flow seem potentially necessary and sufficient because they are based on the knowledge of all variables that may affect the elements of the system.
Physiology	The study of the functions and activities of living cells, tissues, and organs and of the physical and chemical phenomena involved is referred to as physiology.
Auditory nerve	The vestibulocochlear nerve is the eighth of twelve cranial nerves, and also known as the auditory nerve. It is the nerve along which the sensory cells (the hair cells) of the inner ear transmit information to the brain. It consists of the cochlear nerve, carrying information about hearing, and the vestibular nerve, carrying information about balance.
Neuron	The neuron is the primary cell of the nervous system. They are found in the brain, the spinal cord, in the nerves and ganglia of the peripheral nervous system. It is a specialized cell that conducts impulses through the nervous system and contains three major parts: cell body, dendrites, and an axon. It can have many dendrites but only one axon.
Population	Population refers to all members of a well-defined group of organisms, events, or things.
Nerve	A nerve is an enclosed, cable-like bundle of nerve fibers or axons, which includes the glia that ensheath the axons in myelin. Neurons are sometimes called nerve cells, though this term is technically imprecise since many neurons do not form nerves.
Localization of function	Localization of function is the concept that different parts of the brain serve different, specifiable functions in the control of mental experience and behavior.
Right hemisphere	The brain is divided into left and right cerebral hemispheres. The right hemisphere of the cortex controls the left side of the body.
Left hemisphere	The left hemisphere of the cortex controls the right side of the body, coordinates complex movements, and, in 95% of people, controls the production of speech and written language.
Lateralization	Lateralization refers to the dominance of one hemisphere of the brain for specific functions.
Aphasia	Aphasia is a loss or impairment of the ability to produce or comprehend language, due to brain damage. It is usually a result of damage to the language centers of the brain.
Tactile	Pertaining to the sense of touch is referred to as tactile.
Brain imaging	Brain imaging is a fairly recent discipline within medicine and neuroscience. Brain imaging

Chapter 12. Speech Perception

falls into two broad categories -- structural imaging and functional imaging.

Chapter 12. Speech Perception

Chapter 13. The Cutaneous Senses

Evolution	Commonly used to refer to gradual change, evolution is the change in the frequency of alleles within a population from one generation to the next. This change may be caused by different mechanisms, including natural selection, genetic drift, or changes in population (gene flow).
Perception	Perception is the process of acquiring, interpreting, selecting, and organizing sensory information.
Species	Species refers to a reproductively isolated breeding population.
Somatosensory system	Somatosensory system consists of the various sensory receptors that trigger the experiences labelled as touch or pressure, temperature, pain, and the sensations of muscle movement and joint position including posture, movement, and facial expression.
Proprioception	Proprioception is the sense of the position of parts of the body, relative to other neighboring parts of the body.
Sensation	Sensation is the first stage in the chain of biochemical and neurologic events that begins with the impinging of a stimulus upon the receptor cells of a sensory organ, which then leads to perception, the mental state that is reflected in statements like "I see a uniformly blue wall."
Receptor	A sensory receptor is a structure that recognizes a stimulus in the internal or external environment of an organism. In response to stimuli the sensory receptor initiates sensory transduction by creating graded potentials or action potentials in the same cell or in an adjacent one.
Senses	The senses are systems that consist of a sensory cell type that respond to a specific kind of physical energy, and that correspond to a defined region within the brain where the signals are received and interpreted.
Gastrointestnal tract	The gastrointestinal tract is the system of organs within multicellular animals which takes in food, digests it to extract energy and nutrients, and expels the remaining waste.
Lungs	The lungs are the essential organs of respiration. Its principal function is to transport oxygen from the atmosphere into the bloodstream, and excrete carbon dioxide from the bloodstream into the atmosphere.
Mechanoreceptor	A mechanoreceptor is a sensory receptor that responds to mechanical pressure or distortion.
Tactile	Pertaining to the sense of touch is referred to as tactile.
Nerve	A nerve is an enclosed, cable-like bundle of nerve fibers or axons, which includes the glia that ensheath the axons in myelin. Neurons are sometimes called nerve cells, though this term is technically imprecise since many neurons do not form nerves.
Gland	A gland is an organ in an animal's body that synthesizes a substance for release such as hormones, often into the bloodstream or into cavities inside the body or its outer surface.
Psychophysics	Psychophysics refers to the study of the mathematical relationship between the physical aspects of stimuli and our psychological experience of them.
Physiology	The study of the functions and activities of living cells, tissues, and organs and of the physical and chemical phenomena involved is referred to as physiology.
Stimulus	A change in an environmental condition that elicits a response is a stimulus.
Receptive field	The receptive field of a sensory neuron is a region of sensitivity in which the presence of a stimulus will alter the firing of that neuron.
Neuron	The neuron is the primary cell of the nervous system. They are found in the brain, the spinal cord, in the nerves and ganglia of the peripheral nervous system. It is a specialized cell that conducts impulses through the nervous system and contains three major parts: cell body,

Chapter 13. The Cutaneous Senses

Chapter 13. The Cutaneous Senses

	dendrites, and an axon. It can have many dendrites but only one axon.
Threshold	In general, a threshold is a fixed location or value where an abrupt change is observed. In the sensory modalities, it is the minimum amount of stimulus energy necessary to elicit a sensory response.
Graham	Graham has conducted a number of studies that reveal stronger socioeconomic-status influences rather than ethnic influences in achievement.
Nerve impulse	A nerve impulse is a change in the electric potential of a neuron; a wave of depolarization spreads along the neuron and causes the release of a neurotransmitter.
Thermoreceptors	Thermoreceptors are located under the skin, and respond to increases and decreases in temperature.
Retina	The retina is a thin layer of cells at the back of the eyeball. It is the part of the eye which converts light into nervous signals. The retina contains photoreceptor cells which receive the light; the resulting neural signals then undergo complex processing by other neurons of the retina, and are transformed into action potentials in retinal ganglion cells whose axons form the optic nerve.
Fovea	The fovea, a part of the eye, is a spot located in the center of the macula. The fovea is responsible for sharp central vision, which is necessary in humans for reading, watching television or movies, driving, and any activity where visual detail is of primary importance.
Two-point threshold	Two-point threshold is the least distance by which two stimuli touching the skin must be separated before the person will report that there are two stimuli, not one, on 50% of the trials.
Cones	Cones are photoreceptors that transmit sensations of color, function in bright light, and used in visual acuity. Infants prior to months of age can only distinguish green and red indicating the cones are not fully developed; they can see all of the colors by 2 months of
Rods	Rods are cylindrical shaped photoreceptors that are sensitive to the intensity of light. Rods require less light to function than cone cells, and therefore are the primary source of visual information at night.
Brain	The brain controls and coordinates most movement, behavior and homeostatic body functions such as heartbeat, blood pressure, fluid balance and body temperature. Functions of the brain are responsible for cognition, emotion, memory, motor learning and other sorts of learning. The brain is primarily made up of two types of cells: glia and neurons.
Anatomy	Anatomy is the branch of biology that deals with the structure and organization of living things. It can be divided into animal anatomy (zootomy) and plant anatomy (phytonomy). Major branches of anatomy include comparative anatomy, histology, and human anatomy.
Auditory system	The auditory system is the sensory system for the sense of hearing. On its path from the outside world to the forebrain, sound information is preserved and modified in many ways. It changes media twice, first from air to fluid, then from fluid to action potentials.
Large fibers	Large fibers refer to the nerve fibers in the dorsal horns of the spinal cord that regulate the pattern and intensity of pain sensations. They close the gate, decreasing the transmission of painful stimuli.
Spinal cord	The spinal cord is a part of the vertebrate nervous system that is enclosed in and protected by the vertebral column (it passes through the spinal canal). It consists of nerve cells. The spinal cord carries sensory signals and motor innervation to most of the skeletal muscles in the body.
Thalamus	An area near the center of the brain involved in the relay of sensory information to the

Go to Cram101.com for the Practice Tests for this Chapter.

Chapter 13. The Cutaneous Senses

Chapter 13. The Cutaneous Senses

	cortex and in the functions of sleep and attention is the thalamus.
Nucleus	In neuroanatomy, a cluster of cell bodies of neurons within the central nervous system is a nucleus.
Synapse	A synapse is specialized junction through which cells of the nervous system signal to one another and to non-neuronal cells such as muscles or glands.
Right hemisphere	The brain is divided into left and right cerebral hemispheres. The right hemisphere of the cortex controls the left side of the body.
Left hemisphere	The left hemisphere of the cortex controls the right side of the body, coordinates complex movements, and, in 95% of people, controls the production of speech and written language.
Somatosensory cortex	The primary somatosensory cortex is across the central sulcus and behind the primary motor cortex configured to generally correspond with the arrangement of nearby motor cells related to specific body parts. It is the main sensory receptive area for the sense of touch.
Parietal lobe	The parietal lobe is positioned above (superior to) the occipital lobe and behind (posterior to) the frontal lobe. It plays important roles in integrating sensory information from various senses, and in the manipulation of objects.
Somatosensory	Somatosensory system consists of the various sensory receptors that trigger the experiences labelled as touch or pressure, temperature, pain, and the sensations of muscle movement and joint position including posture, movement, and facial expression.
Homunculus	Homunculus is a term used in a number of ways to describe systems that are thought of as being run by a "little man" inside. For instance, the homunculus continues to be considered as one of the major theories on the origin of consciousness, that there is a part in the brain whose purpose is to be "you".
Temporal lobe	The temporal lobe is part of the cerebrum. It lies at the side of the brain, beneath the lateral or Sylvian fissure. Adjacent areas in the superior, posterior and lateral parts of the temporal lobe are involved in high-level auditory processing.
Visual cortex	The visual cortex is the general term applied to both the primary visual cortex and the visual association area. Anatomically, the visual cortex occupies the entire occipital lobe, the inferior temporal lobe (IT), posterior parts of the parietal lobe, and a few small regions in the frontal lobe.
Penfield	Penfield treated patients with severe epilepsy by destroying nerve cells in the brain. Before operating, he stimulated the brain with electrical probes while the patients were conscious on the operating table, and observed their responses. It allowed him to create maps of sensory and motor functions.
Feature detector	A feature detector is sensory system that is highly attuned to a specific stimulus pattern. They are nerve cells in the brain that respond to specific features of the stimulus, such as shape, angle, or movement.
Lateral geniculate nucleus	The lateral geniculate nucleus of the thalamus is a part of the brain, which is the primary processor of visual information, received from the retina, in the CNS.
Adaptation	Adaptation is a lowering of sensitivity to a stimulus following prolonged exposure to that stimulus. Behavioral adaptations are special ways a particular organism behaves to survive in its natural habitat.
Haptic perception	Haptic perception is the ability to acquire information about properties of objects, such as size, weight, and texture, through handling them.
Frontal lobe	The frontal lobe comprises four major folds of cortical tissue: the precentral gyrus,

Chapter 13. The Cutaneous Senses

Chapter 13. The Cutaneous Senses

	superior gyrus and the middle gyrus of the frontal gyri, the inferior frontal gyrus. It has been found to play a part in impulse control, judgement, language, memory, motor function, problem solving, sexual behavior, socialization and spontaneity.
Attention	Attention is the cognitive process of selectively concentrating on one thing while ignoring other things. Psychologists have labeled three types of attention: sustained attention, selective attention, and divided attention.
Pons	The pons is a knob on the brain stem. It is part of the autonomic nervous system, and relays sensory information between the cerebellum and cerebrum. Some theories posit that it has a role in dreaming.
Brain imaging	Brain imaging is a fairly recent discipline within medicine and neuroscience. Brain imaging falls into two broad categories -- structural imaging and functional imaging.
Population	Population refers to all members of a well-defined group of organisms, events, or things.
Motor cortex	Motor cortex refers to the section of cortex that lies in the frontal lobe, just across the central fissure from the sensory cortex. Neural impulses in the motor cortex are linked to muscular responses throughout the body.
Phantom limb	Phantom limb is a feeling that a missing limb is still attached to the body and is moving appropriately with other body parts. Phantom pains can also occur in people who are born without limbs and people who are paralyzed.
Nociceptor	A nociceptor is a sensory receptor that sends signals that cause the perception of pain in response to potentially damaging stimulus. When they are activated, a nociceptor can trigger a reflex.
Cingulate cortex	The part of the limbic system that is believed to process cognitive information in emotion is the cingulate cortex. The cingulate cortex is part of the brain and situated roughly in the middle of the cortex.
Emotion	An emotion is a mental states that arise spontaneously, rather than through conscious effort. They are often accompanied by physiological changes.
Virtual reality	Virtual Reality is an environment that is simulated by a computer. Most virtual reality environments are primarily visual experiences.
Placebo	Placebo refers to a bogus treatment that has the appearance of being genuine.
Control group	A group that does not receive the treatment effect in an experiment is referred to as the control group or sometimes as the comparison group.
Individual differences	Individual differences psychology studies the ways in which individual people differ in their behavior. This is distinguished from other aspects of psychology in that although psychology is ostensibly a study of individuals, modern psychologists invariably study groups.
Gate control theory	The gate control theory of pain, put forward by Ron Melzack and Patrick Wall in 1962, is the idea that pain is not a direct result of activation of pain receptor neurons, but rather its perception is modulated by interaction between different neurons.
Analgesia	Analgesia refers to insensitivity to pain without loss of consciousness.
Endorphin	An endorphin is an endogenous opioid biochemical compound. They are peptides produced by the pituitary gland and the hypothalamus, and they resemble the opiates in their abilities to produce analgesia and a sense of well-being. In other words, they work as "natural pain killers."
Heroin	Heroin is widely and illegally used as a powerful and addictive drug producing intense euphoria, which often disappears with increasing tolerance. Heroin is a semi-synthetic

Chapter 13. The Cutaneous Senses

Chapter 13. The Cutaneous Senses

	opioid. It is the 3,6-diacetyl derivative of morphine and is synthesised from it by acetylation.
Mayer	Mayer developed the concept of emotional intelligence with Peter Salovey. He is one of the authors of the Mayer-Salovey-Caruso Emotional Intelligence Test, and has developed a new, integrated framework for personality psychology, known as the Systems Framework for Pesronality Psychology.
Opium	Opium is a narcotic analgesic drug which is obtained from the unripe seed pods of the opium poppy. Regular use, even for a few days, invariably leads to physical tolerance and dependence. Various degrees of psychological addiction can occur, though this is relatively rare when opioids are properly used..
Neurotransmitter	A neurotransmitter is a chemical that is used to relay, amplify and modulate electrical signals between a neurons and another cell.
Receptor site	A location on the dendrite of a receiving neuron that is tailored to receive a specific neurotransmitter is a receptor site.
Affective	Affective is the way people react emotionally, their ability to feel another living thing's pain or joy.
Affect	A subjective feeling or emotional tone often accompanied by bodily expressions noticeable to others is called affect.
Opiates	A group of narcotics derived from the opium poppy that provide a euphoric rush and depress the nervous system are referred to as opiates.
Visual perception	Visual perception is one of the senses, consisting of the ability to detect light and interpret it. Vision has a specific sensory system.

Chapter 13. The Cutaneous Senses

Chapter 14. The Chemical Senses

Nerve	A nerve is an enclosed, cable-like bundle of nerve fibers or axons, which includes the glia that ensheath the axons in myelin. Neurons are sometimes called nerve cells, though this term is technically imprecise since many neurons do not form nerves.
Perception	Perception is the process of acquiring, interpreting, selecting, and organizing sensory information.
Sensation	Sensation is the first stage in the chain of biochemical and neurologic events that begins with the impinging of a stimulus upon the receptor cells of a sensory organ, which then leads to perception, the mental state that is reflected in statements like "I see a uniformly blue wall."
Olfaction	Olfaction, the sense of odor (smell), is the detection of chemicals dissolved in air. Smells are sensed by the olfactory epithelium located in the nose and processed by the olfactory system.
Receptor	A sensory receptor is a structure that recognizes a stimulus in the internal or external environment of an organism. In response to stimuli the sensory receptor initiates sensory transduction by creating graded potentials or action potentials in the same cell or in an adjacent one.
Senses	The senses are systems that consist of a sensory cell type that respond to a specific kind of physical energy, and that correspond to a defined region within the brain where the signals are received and interpreted.
Neurogenesis	Neurogenesis literally means "birth of neurons". Neurogenesis is most prevalent during pre-natal development and is the process by which neurons are created to populate the growing brain.
Inner ear	The inner ear consists of the oval window, cochlea, and basilar membrane.
Sexual reproduction	Sexual reproduction is a biological process by which organisms create descendants through the combination of genetic material taken randomly and independently from two different members of the species.
Species	Species refers to a reproductively isolated breeding population.
Anosmia	Anosmia is the lack of olfaction, or a loss of the sense of smell. It can be either temporary or permanent.
Olfactory system	The olfactory system is the sensory system used for the sense of smell. The olfactory system is often spoken of along with the gustatory system as the chemosensory senses because both transduce chemical signals into perception
Chemical senses	Chemical senses include smell and taste.
Difference threshold	Difference threshold refers to the minimal difference in intensity required between two sources of energy so that they will be perceived as being different 50 percent of the time.
Variability	Statistically, variability refers to how much the scores in a distribution spread out, away from the mean.
Threshold	In general, a threshold is a fixed location or value where an abrupt change is observed. In the sensory modalities, it is the minimum amount of stimulus energy necessary to elicit a sensory response.
Stimulus	A change in an environmental condition that elicits a response is a stimulus.
Experimental group	Experimental group refers to any group receiving a treatment effect in an experiment.
Control group	A group that does not receive the treatment effect in an experiment is referred to as the

Chapter 14. The Chemical Senses

Chapter 14. The Chemical Senses

	control group or sometimes as the comparison group.
Synchrony	In child development, synchrony is the carefully coordinated interaction between the parent and the child or adolescent in which, often unknowingly, they are attuned to each other's behavior.
Olfactory mucosa	The olfactory mucosa is an organ made up of the olfactory epithelium and the mucosa, or mucus secreting glands, behind the epithelium. The mucus protects the olfactory epithelium and allows odors to dissolve so that they can be detected by olfactory receptor neurons.
Nasal cavity	The nasal cavity is a large air-filled space above and behind the nose in the middle of the face. The nasal cavity is important in warming and cleaning the air as it is inhaled. The nasal cavity also contains organs involved in olfaction.
Transduction	Transduction in the nervous system typically refers to synaptic events wherein an electrical signal, known as an action potential, is converted into a chemical one via the release of neurotransmitters. Conversely, in sensory transduction a chemical or physical stimulus is transduced by sensory receptors into an electrical signal.
Neuron	The neuron is the primary cell of the nervous system. They are found in the brain, the spinal cord, in the nerves and ganglia of the peripheral nervous system. It is a specialized cell that conducts impulses through the nervous system and contains three major parts: cell body, dendrites, and an axon. It can have many dendrites but only one axon.
Olfactory bulb	The olfactory bulb is a part of the brain that is a distinct outgrowth from the forebrain. It plays a major role in olfaction, which is the perception of smells. The olfactory bulb receives direct input from olfactory nerve, made up of the axons from approximately 10 million olfactory receptor neurons in the olfactory mucosa, a region of the nasal cavity.
Ion channel	An Ion channel is a pore-forming protein that help establish the small voltage gradient that exists across the membrane of all living cells, by controlling the flow of ions. They are present in the membranes that surround all biological cells.
Brain	The brain controls and coordinates most movement, behavior and homeostatic body functions such as heartbeat, blood pressure, fluid balance and body temperature. Functions of the brain are responsible for cognition, emotion, memory, motor learning and other sorts of learning. The brain is primarily made up of two types of cells: glia and neurons.
Amino acid	Amino acid is the basic structural building unit of proteins. They form short polymer chains called peptides or polypeptides which in turn form structures called proteins.
Protein	A protein is a complex, high-molecular-weight organic compound that consists of amino acids joined by peptide bonds. It is essential to the structure and function of all living cells and viruses. Many are enzymes or subunits of enzymes.
Olfactory nerve	The olfactory nerve is the first of twelve cranial nerves. It consists of a collection of sensory nerve fibers that extend down from the olfactory bulb and pass through the many openings of the cribriform plate, a sieve-like structure. The specialized olfactory receptor neurons of the olfactory nerve are located in the olfactory mucosa of the upper parts of the nasal cavity.
Axon	An axon, or "nerve fiber," is a long slender projection of a nerve cell, or "neuron," which conducts electrical impulses away from the neuron's cell body or soma.
Ion	An ion is an atom or group of atoms with a net electric charge. The energy required to detach an electron in its lowest energy state from an atom or molecule of a gas with less net electric charge is called the ionization potential, or ionization energy.
Glomeruli	Glomeruli are important waystations in the pathway from the nose to the olfactory cortex. Each receives input from olfactory receptor neurons expressing only one type of olfactory

Chapter 14. The Chemical Senses

Chapter 14. The Chemical Senses

	receptor. There are tens of millions of olfactory receptor cells, but only about two thousand glomeruli. By combining so much input, the olfactory system is able to detect even very faint odors.
Synapse	A synapse is specialized junction through which cells of the nervous system signal to one another and to non-neuronal cells such as muscles or glands.
Visual cortex	The visual cortex is the general term applied to both the primary visual cortex and the visual association area. Anatomically, the visual cortex occupies the entire occipital lobe, the inferior temporal lobe (IT), posterior parts of the parietal lobe, and a few small regions in the frontal lobe.
Frontal lobe	The frontal lobe comprises four major folds of cortical tissue: the precentral gyrus, superior gyrus and the middle gyrus of the frontal gyri, the inferior frontal gyrus. It has been found to play a part in impulse control, judgement, language, memory, motor function, problem solving, sexual behavior, socialization and spontaneity.
Temporal lobe	The temporal lobe is part of the cerebrum. It lies at the side of the brain, beneath the lateral or Sylvian fissure. Adjacent areas in the superior, posterior and lateral parts of the temporal lobe are involved in high-level auditory processing.
Cerebral cortex	The cerebral cortex is the outermost layer of the cerebrum and has a grey color. It is made up of four lobes and it is involved in many complex brain functions including memory, perceptual awareness, "thinking", language and consciousness. The cerebral cortex receives sensory information from many different sensory organs eg: eyes, ears, etc. and processes the information.
Amygdala	Located in the brain's medial temporal lobe, the almond-shaped amygdala is believed to play a key role in the emotions. It forms part of the limbic system and is linked to both fear responses and pleasure. Its size is positively correlated with aggressive behavior across species.
Anatomy	Anatomy is the branch of biology that deals with the structure and organization of living things. It can be divided into animal anatomy (zootomy) and plant anatomy (phytonomy). Major branches of anatomy include comparative anatomy, histology, and human anatomy.
Papillae	The bumps on the tongue that contain taste buds, the receptors for taste, are papillae.
Cones	Cones are photoreceptors that transmit sensations of color, function in bright light, and used in visual acuity. Infants prior to months of age can only distinguish green and red indicating the cones are not fully developed; they can see all of the colors by 2 months of
Receptor site	A location on the dendrite of a receiving neuron that is tailored to receive a specific neurotransmitter is a receptor site.
Taste bud	The taste bud (or lingual papillae) is a small structure on the upper surface of the tongue that provides information about the taste of food being eaten. It is known that there are five taste sensations: Sweet, Bitter, Umami, Salty and Sour.
Affect	A subjective feeling or emotional tone often accompanied by bodily expressions noticeable to others is called affect.
Glossopharyngeal nerve	The glossopharyngeal nerve is the ninth of twelve cranial nerves. It exits the brainstem out from the sides of the upper medulla, just rostral (closer to the nose) to the vagus nerve. It receives sensory fibers from the posterior 1/3 of the tongue, the tonsils, the pharynx, the middle ear and the carotid body.
Vagus nerve	The vagus nerve is tenth of twelve paired cranial nerves and is the only nerve that starts in the brainstem (somewhere in the medulla oblongata) and extends all the way down past the head, right down to the abdomen. The vagus nerve is arguably the single most important nerve

Go to Cram101.com for the Practice Tests for this Chapter.

Chapter 14. The Chemical Senses

Chapter 14. The Chemical Senses

	in the body.
Larynx	The larynx, or voicebox, is an organ in the neck of mammals involved in protection of the trachea and sound production. The larynx houses the vocal cords, and is situated at the point where the upper tract splits into the trachea and the esophagus.
Brain stem	The brain stem is the stalk of the brain below the cerebral hemispheres. It is the major route for communication between the forebrain and the spinal cord and peripheral nerves. It also controls various functions including respiration, regulation of heart rhythms, and primary aspects of sound localization.
Thalamus	An area near the center of the brain involved in the relay of sensory information to the cortex and in the functions of sleep and attention is the thalamus.
Nucleus	In neuroanatomy, a cluster of cell bodies of neurons within the central nervous system is a nucleus.
Glutamate	Glutamate is one of the 20 standard amino acids used by all organisms in their proteins. It is critical for proper cell function, but it is not an essential nutrient in humans because it can be manufactured from other compounds.
Magnitude estimation	Magnitude estimation involves subjects attempting to report numerically the perceived intensity of sensation relative to a standard, where the standard is ascribed a specific numeric value either by the experimenter or subject.
Reflection	Reflection is the process of rephrasing or repeating thoughts and feelings expressed, making the person more aware of what they are saying or thinking.
Coding	In senation, coding is the process by which information about the quality and quantity of a stimulus is preserved in the pattern of action potentials sent through sensory neurons to the central nervous system.
Hypothesis	A specific statement about behavior or mental processes that is testable through research is a hypothesis.
Deprivation	Deprivation, is the loss or withholding of normal stimulation, nutrition, comfort, love, and so forth; a condition of lacking. The level of stimulation is less than what is required.
Basic research	Basic research has as its primary objective the advancement of knowledge and the theoretical understanding of the relations among variables . It is exploratory and often driven by the researcher's curiosity, interest or hunch.
Tactile	Pertaining to the sense of touch is referred to as tactile.
Glucose	Glucose, a simple monosaccharide sugar, is one of the most important carbohydrates and is used as a source of energy in animals and plants. Glucose is one of the main products of photosynthesis and starts respiration.
Satiety	Satiety refers to the state of being satisfied; fullness.
Physiology	The study of the functions and activities of living cells, tissues, and organs and of the physical and chemical phenomena involved is referred to as physiology.
Somatosensory cortex	The primary somatosensory cortex is across the central sulcus and behind the primary motor cortex configured to generally correspond with the arrangement of nearby motor cells related to specific body parts. It is the main sensory receptive area for the sense of touch.
Learning	Learning is a relatively permanent change in behavior that results from experience. Thus, to attribute a behavioral change to learning, the change must be relatively permanent and must result from experience.
Plasticity	The capacity for modification and change is referred to as plasticity.

Chapter 14. The Chemical Senses

Chapter 14. The Chemical Senses

Go to **Cram101.com** for the Practice Tests for this Chapter.

Chapter 14. The Chemical Senses

Chapter 15. Perceptual Development

Attention	Attention is the cognitive process of selectively concentrating on one thing while ignoring other things. Psychologists have labeled three types of attention: sustained attention, selective attention, and divided attention.
Perception	Perception is the process of acquiring, interpreting, selecting, and organizing sensory information.
Stimulus	A change in an environmental condition that elicits a response is a stimulus.
Homogeneous	In biology homogeneous has a meaning similar to its meaning in mathematics. Generally it means "the same" or "of the same quality or general property".
Habituation	In habituation there is a progressive reduction in the response probability with continued repetition of a stimulus.
Visual acuity	Visual acuity is the eye's ability to detect fine details and is the quantitative measure of the eye's ability to see an in-focus image at a certain distance.
Visual cortex	The visual cortex is the general term applied to both the primary visual cortex and the visual association area. Anatomically, the visual cortex occupies the entire occipital lobe, the inferior temporal lobe (IT), posterior parts of the parietal lobe, and a few small regions in the frontal lobe.
Electrode	Any device used to electrically stimulate nerve tissue or to record its activity is an electrode.
Neuron	The neuron is the primary cell of the nervous system. They are found in the brain, the spinal cord, in the nerves and ganglia of the peripheral nervous system. It is a specialized cell that conducts impulses through the nervous system and contains three major parts: cell body, dendrites, and an axon. It can have many dendrites but only one axon.
Dishabituation	A renewed interest in a stimulus is referred to as dishabituation.
Receptor	A sensory receptor is a structure that recognizes a stimulus in the internal or external environment of an organism. In response to stimuli the sensory receptor initiates sensory transduction by creating graded potentials or action potentials in the same cell or in an adjacent one.
Retina	The retina is a thin layer of cells at the back of the eyeball. It is the part of the eye which converts light into nervous signals. The retina contains photoreceptor cells which receive the light; the resulting neural signals then undergo complex processing by other neurons of the retina, and are transformed into action potentials in retinal ganglion cells whose axons form the optic nerve.
Cones	Cones are photoreceptors that transmit sensations of color, function in bright light, and used in visual acuity. Infants prior to months of age can only distinguish green and red indicating the cones are not fully developed; they can see all of the colors by 2 months of
Fovea	The fovea, a part of the eye, is a spot located in the center of the macula. The fovea is responsible for sharp central vision, which is necessary in humans for reading, watching television or movies, driving, and any activity where visual detail is of primary importance.
Law of similarity	The law of similarity states if two things are similar, the thought of one will tend to trigger the thought of the other. It is a principle of Gestalt organization in which similar stimuli are percieved as belonging together as a unit.
Rods	Rods are cylindrical shaped photoreceptors that are sensitive to the intensity of light. Rods require less light to function than cone cells, and therefore are the primary source of visual information at night.
Inference	Inference is the act or process of drawing a conclusion based solely on what one already

Chapter 15. Perceptual Development

Chapter 15. Perceptual Development

	knows.
Discrimination	In Learning theory, discrimination refers the ability to distinguish between a conditioned stimulus and other stimuli. It can be brought about by extensive training or differential reinforcement. In social terms, it is the denial of privileges to a person or a group on the basis of prejudice.
Brightness	The dimension of visual sensation that is dependent on the intensity of light reflected from a surface and that corresponds to the amplitude of the light wave is called brightness.
Trichromat	A trichromat is an organism for which the perceptual effect of any chosen light from its visible spectrum can be matched by a mixture of no more than three different pure spectral lights. The organism's retina contains three types of color receptors with different absorption spectra.
Pictorial depth cues	Clues about distance that can be given in a flat picture are pictorial depth cues. They operate on real scenes and when viewing pictures. They include occlusion, relative image size for familiar objects, linear perspective, texture gradient, differential lighting of surfaces, and position relative location.
Binocular disparity	A binocular depth cue resulting from differences between the two retinal images formed of an object viewed at distances up to about 20 feet is referred to as binocular disparity.
Fixation	Fixation in abnormal psychology is the state where an individual becomes obsessed with an attachment to another human, animal or inanimate object. Fixation in vision refers to maintaining the gaze in a constant direction. .
Stereopsis	Stereopsis is the process in visual perception leading to perception of the depth or distance of objects. Depth from stereopsis arises from the slightly different positions each eye occupies on the head, a form of parallax.
Premise	A premise is a statement presumed true within the context of a discourse, especially of a logical argument.
Occlusion	The monocular depth cue occlusion is the blocking of sight of objects by other objects. It creates a "ranking" of nearness, and does not give any insight as to actual distances. In the absence of color or binocular vision, it often serves as the method of last resort for rudimentary depth perception.
Chemical senses	Chemical senses include smell and taste.
Texture gradient	Texture gradient is a monocular cue for depth based on the perception that closer objects appear to have rougher surfaces. Objects appear denser as they go further away.
Intonation	The use of pitches of varying levels to help communicate meaning is called intonation.
Fetus	A fetus develops from the end of the 8th week of pregnancy (when the major structures have formed), until birth.
Threshold	In general, a threshold is a fixed location or value where an abrupt change is observed. In the sensory modalities, it is the minimum amount of stimulus energy necessary to elicit a sensory response.
Sound localization	Sound localization is a listener's ability to identify the location of origin of a detected sound. There are two general methods for sound localization, binaural cues and monaural cues.
Darwin	Darwin achieved lasting fame as originator of the theory of evolution through natural selection. His book Expression of Emotions in Man and Animals is generally considered the first text on comparative psychology.
Conditioning	Conditioning describes the process by which behaviors can be learned or modified through

Chapter 15. Perceptual Development

Chapter 15. Perceptual Development

	interaction with the environment.
Affect	A subjective feeling or emotional tone often accompanied by bodily expressions noticeable to others is called affect.
Learning	Learning is a relatively permanent change in behavior that results from experience. Thus, to attribute a behavioral change to learning, the change must be relatively permanent and must result from experience.
Olfaction	Olfaction, the sense of odor (smell), is the detection of chemicals dissolved in air. Smells are sensed by the olfactory epithelium located in the nose and processed by the olfactory system.
Senses	The senses are systems that consist of a sensory cell type that respond to a specific kind of physical energy, and that correspond to a defined region within the brain where the signals are received and interpreted.
Intermodal matching	Intermodal matching is the ability to recognize an object in one sensory or cognitive modality as the same object in another modality.
Plasticity	The capacity for modification and change is referred to as plasticity.
Depth cues	Perceptual features that impart information about distance and three-dimensional space are called depth cues.
Myopia	Myopia is a refractive defect of the eye in which light focuses in front of the retina. Those with myopia are often described as nearsighted or short-sighted in that they typically can see nearby objects clearly but distant objects appear blurred because the lens cannot flatten enough.
Hyperopia	Hyperopia is a defect of vision caused by an imperfection in the eye (often when the eyeball is too short or when the lens cannot become round enough), causing inability to focus on near objects, and in extreme cases causing a sufferer to be unable to focus on objects at any distance.
Feedback	Feedback refers to information returned to a person about the effects a response has had.
Intermodal perception	The ability to relate and integrate information about two or more sensory modalities, such as vision and hearing, is referred to as intermodal perception.

Chapter 15. Perceptual Development

Chapter 16. Clinical Aspects of Vision and Hearing

Sensorineural hearing loss	Sensorineural hearing loss is a type of hearing loss in which the root cause lies in the vestibulocochlear nerve (Cranial nerve VIII), the inner ear, cochlea, or central processing centers of the brain.
Conductive hearing loss	Conductive hearing loss is a failure in the efficient conduction of sound waves through the outer ear, typanic membrane (eardrum) or middle ears (ossicles). This type of hearing loss may occur in conjunction with sensorineural hearing loss or alone.
Retina	The retina is a thin layer of cells at the back of the eyeball. It is the part of the eye which converts light into nervous signals. The retina contains photoreceptor cells which receive the light; the resulting neural signals then undergo complex processing by other neurons of the retina, and are transformed into action potentials in retinal ganglion cells whose axons form the optic nerve.
Cornea	The cornea is the transparent front part of the eye that covers the iris, pupil, and anterior chamber and provides most of an eye's optical power. Together with the lens, the cornea refracts light and consequently helps the eye to focus.
Optic nerve	The optic nerve is the nerve that transmits visual information from the retina to the brain. The optic nerve is composed of retinal ganglion cell axons and support cells.
Glaucoma	Glaucoma is a group of diseases of the optic nerve involving loss of retinal ganglion cells. Untreated glaucoma leads to permanent damage of the optic nerve and resultant visual field loss, which can progress to blindness.
Tumor	A tumor is an abnormal growth that when located in the brain can either be malignant and directly destroy brain tissue, or be benign and disrupt functioning by increasing intracranial pressure.
Nearsightedness	A vision deficiency in which close objects are seen clearly but distant objects appear blurry is nearsightedness.
Myopia	Myopia is a refractive defect of the eye in which light focuses in front of the retina. Those with myopia are often described as nearsighted or short-sighted in that they typically can see nearby objects clearly but distant objects appear blurred because the lens cannot flatten enough.
Affect	A subjective feeling or emotional tone often accompanied by bodily expressions noticeable to others is called affect.
Farsightedness	Hyperopia, also known as farsightedness, is a defect of vision caused by an imperfection in the eye (often when the eyeball is too short), causing inability to focus on near objects, and in extreme cases causing a sufferer to be unable to focus on objects at any distance.
Hyperopia	Hyperopia is a defect of vision caused by an imperfection in the eye (often when the eyeball is too short or when the lens cannot become round enough), causing inability to focus on near objects, and in extreme cases causing a sufferer to be unable to focus on objects at any distance.
Accommodation	Piaget's developmental process of accommodation is the modification of currently held schemes or new schemes so that new information inconsistent with the existing schemes can be integrated and understood.
Astigmatism	Astigmatism is a refraction error of the eye characterized by an aspherical cornea in which one axis of corneal steepness is greater than the perpendicular axis.
Visual acuity	Visual acuity is the eye's ability to detect fine details and is the quantitative measure of the eye's ability to see an in-focus image at a certain distance.
Peripheral	Peripheral vision is that part of vision that occurs outside the very center of gaze.

Go to Cram101.com for the Practice Tests for this Chapter.

Chapter 16. Clinical Aspects of Vision and Hearing

Chapter 16. Clinical Aspects of Vision and Hearing

vision	Peripheral vision is weak in humans, especially at distinguishing color and shape. This is because the density of receptor cells on the retina is greatest at the center and lowest at the edges
Fovea	The fovea, a part of the eye, is a spot located in the center of the macula. The fovea is responsible for sharp central vision, which is necessary in humans for reading, watching television or movies, driving, and any activity where visual detail is of primary importance.
Iris	The iris is the most visible part of the eye. The iris is an annulus (or flattened ring) consisting of pigmented fibrovascular tissue known as a stroma. The stroma connects a sphincter muscle, which contracts the pupil, and a set of dialator muscles which open it.
Congenital	A condition existing at birth is referred to as congenital.
Cataracts	A cataract is any opacity which develops in the crystalline lens of the eye or in its envelope. Cataracts form for a variety of reasons, including long term ultraviolet exposure, secondary effects of diseases such as diabetes, or simply due to advanced age.
Ultrasound	Ultrasound is sound with a frequency greater than the upper limit of human hearing, approximately 20 kilohertz. Medical use can visualise muscle and soft tissue, making them useful for scanning the organs, and obstetric ultrasonography is commonly used during pregnancy.
Perception	Perception is the process of acquiring, interpreting, selecting, and organizing sensory information.
Brain	The brain controls and coordinates most movement, behavior and homeostatic body functions such as heartbeat, blood pressure, fluid balance and body temperature. Functions of the brain are responsible for cognition, emotion, memory, motor learning and other sorts of learning. The brain is primarily made up of two types of cells: glia and neurons.
Epithelium	Epithelium is a tissue composed of a layer of cells. Epithelium can be found lining internal or external (e.g. skin) free surfaces of the body. Functions of epithelial cells include secretion, absorption and protection.
Pupil	In the eye, the pupil is the opening in the middle of the iris. It appears black because most of the light entering it is absorbed by the tissues inside the eye. The size of the pupil is controlled by involuntary contraction and dilation of the iris, in order to regulate the intensity of light entering the eye. This is known as the pupillary reflex.
Life expectancy	The number of years that will probably be lived by the average person born in a particular year is called life expectancy.
Diabetes	Diabetes is a medical disorder characterized by varying or persistent elevated blood sugar levels, especially after eating. All types of diabetes share similar symptoms and complications at advanced stages: dehydration and ketoacidosis, cardiovascular disease, chronic renal failure, retinal damage which can lead to blindness, nerve damage which can lead to erectile dysfunction, gangrene with risk of amputation of toes, feet, and even legs.
Vitreous humor	Vitreous humor is the clear aqueous solution that fills the space between the lens and the retina of the vertebrate eyeball. The primary purpose to provide a cushioned support for the rest of the eye, as well as a clear unobstructed path for light to travel to the retina.
Stages	Stages represent relatively discrete periods of time in which functioning is qualitatively different from functioning at other periods.
Macular degeneration	Macular degeneration is a medical condition where the light sensing cells in the macula malfunction and over time cease to work.
Macula	The macula is an oval yellow spot near the center of the retina of the human eye. Near its

Chapter 16. Clinical Aspects of Vision and Hearing

Chapter 16. Clinical Aspects of Vision and Hearing

	center is the fovea, a small pit that contains the largest concentration of cone cells in the eye and is responsible for central vision.
Receptor	A sensory receptor is a structure that recognizes a stimulus in the internal or external environment of an organism. In response to stimuli the sensory receptor initiates sensory transduction by creating graded potentials or action potentials in the same cell or in an adjacent one.
Enzyme	An enzyme is a protein that catalyzes, or speeds up, a chemical reaction. Enzymes are essential to sustain life because most chemical reactions in biological cells would occur too slowly, or would lead to different products, without enzymes.
Anchor	An anchor is a sample of work or performance used to set the specific performance standard for a rubric level .
Hypothesis	A specific statement about behavior or mental processes that is testable through research is a hypothesis.
Adolescence	The period of life bounded by puberty and the assumption of adult responsibilities is adolescence.
Nerve impulse	A nerve impulse is a change in the electric potential of a neuron; a wave of depolarization spreads along the neuron and causes the release of a neurotransmitter.
Nerve	A nerve is an enclosed, cable-like bundle of nerve fibers or axons, which includes the glia that ensheath the axons in myelin. Neurons are sometimes called nerve cells, though this term is technically imprecise since many neurons do not form nerves.
Aqueous humor	The aqueous humor is the clear, watery fluid that fills the complex space in the front of the eye which is bounded at the front by the cornea and at the rear by the front surface or face of the vitreous humor.
Blocking	If the one of the two members of a compound stimulus fails to produce the CR due to an earlier conditioning of the other member of the compound stimulus, blocking has occurred.
Presbyopia	Presbyopia is the eye's diminished power of accommodation that occurs with aging. Presbyopia is not a disease as such, but a condition that affects everyone at a certain age.
Ciliary muscle	The ciliary muscle is a smooth muscle that affects zonules in the eye (fibers that suspend the lens in position during accommodation), enabling changes in lens shape for light focusing.
Ophthalmoscope	In 1851, Helmholtz invented the ophthalmoscope, an instrument which can be used to look into the human eye.
Helmholtz	Helmholtz a pioneer of the new science of psychology, was a rigorous experimental physiologist and philospher. He gave us the distinction between sensation and peception and is well known for his theories of color perception and hearing.
Ganglion cell	A ganglion cell is a type of neuron located in the retina of the eye that receives visual information from photoreceptors via various intermediate cells such as bipolar cells, amacrine cells, and horizontal cells. Retinal ganglion cells' axons are myelinated.
Optic disk	The optic disk refers to a hole in the retina where the optic nerve fibers exit the eye. It corresponds to the blind spot.
Stimulus	A change in an environmental condition that elicits a response is a stimulus.
Auditory system	The auditory system is the sensory system for the sense of hearing. On its path from the outside world to the forebrain, sound information is preserved and modified in many ways. It changes media twice, first from air to fluid, then from fluid to action potentials.

Go to **Cram101.com** for the Practice Tests for this Chapter.

Chapter 16. Clinical Aspects of Vision and Hearing

Chapter 16. Clinical Aspects of Vision and Hearing

Middle ear	The middle ear consists of the eardrum, hammer, anvil, and stirrup.
Outer ear	Outer ear consists of the pinna and the external auditory canal.
Hair cells	Hair cells are the sensory cells of both the auditory system and the vestibular system. The auditory hair cells are located within the organ of Corti on a thin basilar membrane in the cochlea of the inner ear.
Auditory nerve	The vestibulocochlear nerve is the eighth of twelve cranial nerves, and also known as the auditory nerve. It is the nerve along which the sensory cells (the hair cells) of the inner ear transmit information to the brain. It consists of the cochlear nerve, carrying information about hearing, and the vestibular nerve, carrying information about balance.
Cochlea	The Cochlea is the bony tube that contains the basilar membrane and the organ of Corti. The cochlea consists of three fluid-filled chambers - scala tympani and scala vestibuli and scala media.
Tympanic membrane	The tympanic membrane, colloquially known as eardrum, is a thin membrane that separates the outer ear from the middle ear. Its function is to transmit sound from the air to the ossicles inside the middle ear.
Ossicles	The ossicles are the three smallest bones in the human body. They are contained within the middle ear space and serve to transmit sounds from the air to the fluid filled labyrinth (cochlea).
Inner ear	The inner ear consists of the oval window, cochlea, and basilar membrane.
Stapes	The stapes or stirrup is the stirrup-shaped small bone or ossicle in the middle ear which attaches the incus to the fenestra ovalis, the "oval window" which is adjacent to the vestibule of the inner ear. It is the smallest bone in the human body.
Organ of Corti	The Organ of Corti is the hearing organ of the inner ear. It contains receptors that respond to vibrations in the basilar membrane which are caused by sound.
Sensation	Sensation is the first stage in the chain of biochemical and neurologic events that begins with the impinging of a stimulus upon the receptor cells of a sensory organ, which then leads to perception, the mental state that is reflected in statements like "I see a uniformly blue wall."
Suicide	Suicide behavior is rare in childhood but escalates in adolescence. The suicide rate increases in a linear fashion from adolescence through late adulthood.
Bone conduction	Bone conduction is the conduction of sound to the inner ear through the bones of the skull.
Threshold	In general, a threshold is a fixed location or value where an abrupt change is observed. In the sensory modalities, it is the minimum amount of stimulus energy necessary to elicit a sensory response.
Reflex	A simple, involuntary response to a stimulus is referred to as reflex. Reflex actions originate at the spinal cord rather than the brain.
Cochlear implant	A cochlear implant is a hearing device that can help people with certain kinds of hearing impairment or who have a severe to profound hearing loss. The implant works by using the tonotopic organization of the basilar membrane of the inner ear.
Electrode	Any device used to electrically stimulate nerve tissue or to record its activity is an electrode.
McDougall	McDougall was important in the development of the theory of instinct and of social psychology. Opposing behaviorism, he argued that behavior was generally goal-oriented and purposive, an approach he called hormic psychology; in the theory of motivation he held that

Go to **Cram101.com** for the Practice Tests for this Chapter.

Chapter 16. Clinical Aspects of Vision and Hearing

Chapter 16. Clinical Aspects of Vision and Hearing

	individuals are motivated by a significant number of inherited instincts so they might not always understand their own goals.
Basic research	Basic research has as its primary objective the advancement of knowledge and the theoretical understanding of the relations among variables . It is exploratory and often driven by the researcher's curiosity, interest or hunch.
Physiology	The study of the functions and activities of living cells, tissues, and organs and of the physical and chemical phenomena involved is referred to as physiology.
Neuron	The neuron is the primary cell of the nervous system. They are found in the brain, the spinal cord, in the nerves and ganglia of the peripheral nervous system. It is a specialized cell that conducts impulses through the nervous system and contains three major parts: cell body, dendrites, and an axon. It can have many dendrites but only one axon.
Attention	Attention is the cognitive process of selectively concentrating on one thing while ignoring other things. Psychologists have labeled three types of attention: sustained attention, selective attention, and divided attention.
Senses	The senses are systems that consist of a sensory cell type that respond to a specific kind of physical energy, and that correspond to a defined region within the brain where the signals are received and interpreted.
Otitis media	Otitis media refers to infection of the middle ear, an extremely common childhood problem; the attendant temporary or chronic hearing loss may lead to language development delays.
Plasticity	The capacity for modification and change is referred to as plasticity.
Visual cortex	The visual cortex is the general term applied to both the primary visual cortex and the visual association area. Anatomically, the visual cortex occupies the entire occipital lobe, the inferior temporal lobe (IT), posterior parts of the parietal lobe, and a few small regions in the frontal lobe.

Chapter 16. Clinical Aspects of Vision and Hearing

Printed in the United Kingdom
by Lightning Source UK Ltd.
114482UKS00001B/23-24